BAD MOVES

BAD
MOVES

How decision making
goes wrong, and the ethics
of smart drugs

BARBARA J. SAHAKIAN AND
JAMIE NICOLE LABUZETTA

OXFORD
UNIVERSITY PRESS

OXFORD
UNIVERSITY PRESS

Great Clarendon Street, Oxford, OX2 6DP,
United Kingdom

Oxford University Press is a department of the University of Oxford.
It furthers the University's objective of excellence in research, scholarship,
and education by publishing worldwide. Oxford is a registered trade mark of
Oxford University Press in the UK and in certain other countries

© Barbara J. Sahakian and Jamie Nicole LaBuzetta 2013

The moral rights of the authors have been asserted

First Edition published in 2013

Impression: 1

British Library Cataloguing in Publication Data
Data available

Library of Congress Cataloging in Publication Data
Data available

ISBN 978–0–19–966847–2

Printed in Great Britain by
Clays Ltd, St Ives plc

This book is dedicated to all participants who have given their time to assist in neuroscientific and mental health research 'in the name of science'—our understanding of the human mind and development of effective treatments could not move forward without you.

Barbara Sahakian also dedicates this book to her daughters Jacqueline and Miranda Robbins, who have shown a great interest in engaging the public in science and neuroethics.

TABLE OF CONTENTS

PREFACE

Begin at the beginning ... and go on till you come to the end: then stop.
Lewis Carroll, author

The bridges and murky water of the River Cam form the backdrop of the yearly University of Cambridge Science Festival—part of National Science Week in England. Ordinarily, the lecture theatres at the New Museum site in the Cambridge city centre would be filled with sleepy-eyed students sipping coffee, presided over by some extraordinary and eccentric lecturer discussing the role of snail neurons, the nervous system of the *C. elegans* worm, or some other admittedly fascinating but equally esoteric topic. But for one week each spring, the students are let loose, and interested members of the public gather for whatever topics await.

The University of Cambridge Science Festival is an ongoing effort originally intended to make members of the public more aware of cutting-edge scientific advances in fascinating topics such as space exploration, computer technology, composite materials, and the brain. It has developed into a stimulating and successful annual meeting of academics, Cambridge students, professionals, parents, and children, and includes lectures, debates, and interactive programmes for all ages.[1]

Throughout recent years, one recurring theme has been interspersed among others: the science of brain function ('cognition'), and more specifically, the science that illuminates how brain function usually works, how it can go wrong, and how it can be improved. A decade ago, Barbara gave her first Science Week talk on the brain basis of extreme emotions and behaviour—i.e. the ways in which emotions can affect our decision making and make us behave in risky or bizarre ways. Since then, further research has shown that new drugs can produce remarkable effects on patients with certain neurological and psychiatric conditions—conditions that cause them to have trouble making decisions. Even more exciting, and rather more controversial, is the effect that these same medications have on healthy individuals; in some cases, they seem to provide a cognitive 'boost', and have therefore earned the nickname 'smart drugs'. This book is an attempt to expand some of these topics and explain the groundbreaking work currently being done in the areas of decision making, the ways in which normal brain function sometimes fails, the interventions we can employ to 'normalize' abnormal brain behaviour, and the ethical implications raised by some of the smart drugs that are currently available.

A scant mile away from another murky river in the other, younger, Cambridge (across The Pond) you can find the Warren Anatomical Museum at Harvard's Countway Library of Medicine.[2] This library houses a famous skull that features a shattered cheekbone, mangled eye socket, and a large hole at the top. It is the skull of Mr Phineas Gage, who was unfortunate enough to have a metre-long iron rod shoot through his face, the front part of his brain, and out the top of his head.[3] You'll be unsurprised to hear that Gage suffered some brain damage as a result of his accident.[4] Gage has become famous not only for his unlikely survival, but because of the ways in which his personality and cognitive functioning were forever changed by the damage to his brain.[5] These changes led scientists to suspect that specific parts of the brain could be associated with specific behaviours, capabilities, and emotions.

Therefore, Phineas Gage's melancholy story can fairly be said to have sparked a new field of scientific inquiry—quite unintentionally, of course. Before his accident, the various roles of the frontal brain were largely unknown. In fact, many early 19th-century scientists suspected that the frontal area of the brain did not have a specific function.

In the last fifty years, advancements in technology have allowed us to develop tools precise enough to explore the inner workings of the human brain. Without such a technological revolution, we would likely still be theorizing and asking very basic questions about brain function and its relationship to behaviour. But modern tools have allowed us to affirm some basic tenets of neuroscience and answer curious uncertainties about functionality, such as which areas of the brain are activated when a person is trying to remember something, count, move, or is sexually aroused.

Using these tools, researchers have been able to reveal that particular areas of the brain are associated with particular abilities, that errors in function in certain areas of the brain can lead to specific deficits in cognition and, more interestingly, that therapies and drugs can sometimes improve function and improve—or even restore—certain deficient cognitive abilities.

Within the neurosciences, the discipline of neuroethics has also recently exploded, because as progress is made and technological advances allow ever more precise discoveries, we are constantly confronted with previously unimaginable ethical dilemmas. Surely, it is imperative that the students and practitioners of neuroscience discuss these issues [1]; however, some of these topics affect society in such important ways that a wider social discussion is prudent as well. For instance, brain imaging intrigues many patients, and it is increasingly common for patients to ask their physicians to order brain imaging so as to *be certain* there isn't a problem. However, what should one do if something *abnormal*—but not necessarily harmful—is discovered on brain imaging [2]? The topic of these *incidentalomas* is one that is ethically fraught and impinges on many other topics such as healthcare costs, physician autonomy, the roles of insurers and researchers, medical over-treatment, and personal freedom of choice—issues that are active in contemporary society in the United States, the United Kingdom, and elsewhere. Another fraught question—and the one that we will concern ourselves with in this book—is this: What is the proper role for medications that can potentially improve brain function beyond natural limits, so-called *smart drugs*?

The first step towards a productive discussion of these drugs is to understand what they are and what they can do. Therefore, our approach will be to briefly discuss the basics of what we currently know about one aspect of cognition, namely decision making. We will then introduce how decision making goes wrong in certain patient populations, and discuss treatments, including drugs, that can improve it. We use decision making as a conduit because the research that has been done in our lab has largely focused on how certain patient populations make their decisions, and because decision making is an important aspect of the overall cognitive function that determines our life choices. Throughout this book, it should be remembered that decision making is discussed as just *one aspect* of the brain function that is affected by smart drugs—it is a quantifiable component of a much more complicated and subtle process. But for that reason, it can also be a window into the complex role of cognitive therapies in a broader sense. In other words, the significance of smart drugs on decision making is a miniature of the significance of smart drugs on cognitive function more generally. These drugs already exist, and, as we will show, their use is surprisingly widespread. Yet many people have not thought about their potential impact. We hope that this book will be a first step towards a broader understanding of and a broader discussion of the role these drugs have in society. The questions relating to how smart drugs should be used—who should benefit, who should decide, and who should pay—form one of the most important and timely ethical dilemmas in the field of neurosciences today.

1

LIFE CHOICES

Choose life. Choose a job... Choose a starter home. Choose your friends. Choose leisure wear and matching luggage... Choose your future... But why would I want to do a thing like that?   Tagline from the movie *Trainspotting*, 1996

Making good decisions is a crucial skill at every level.   Peter Drucker, educator

Imagine yourself on a Sunday afternoon in summer, sitting on the patio enjoying a drink. It's not quite time to prepare supper, so you take a moment to relax, but your reverie is broken when you realize that your neighbour has wandered into your garden and is masturbating among the roses. You are aghast—scandalous! You then recall that at a dinner party earlier in the month, the same neighbour had grabbed the steak off the host's plate because it looked larger than his own. Your neighbour's spouse immediately runs over and is very apologetic, but you are just left wondering *what on earth is going on.*

What you do not know is that your neighbour has been diagnosed with frontotemporal dementia, an uncommon—but not entirely rare—condition characterized by impulsive behaviour, difficulties with decision making, personality changes, and, eventually, changes in memory and language function. All these changes proceed from altered function in a region of the brain towards the front ('frontal') and side ('temporal') of the head.

The first symptom for most individuals with frontotemporal dementia (FTD) is usually a change in personality. These patients can become impulsive or irritable, withdrawn, childish, and occasionally aggressive. As with our neighbour above, sometimes they become extraordinarily hypersexual, flirt inappropriately, perform lewd behaviours in public, or touch others in an inappropriate manner. Moreover, decisions we take for granted are often very difficult for these patients. For example, they may not be able to decide what to wear in the morning, and *decide* to wear either clothing that is improper or maybe no clothing at all. Family members also report that these patients display poor judgement in various matters. They may run up considerable debt after purchasing things that are unnecessary or extravagant, and sufferers of FTD usually drive very dangerously. Their problems with decision making are due to specific, measurable changes in brain function in particular areas of the brain. These patients make impulsive, risky decisions, but they cannot help it. Caregivers may find this very difficult to keep in mind if much of their time is spent begging collection agencies to forgive debts, apologizing to strangers when the patient behaves inappropriately, and resolving the chaos these individuals can create. As these patients demonstrate for us, a physiological deficit can impair good decision making, which can in turn manifest as quite dramatic and disruptive changes in behaviour.

Frontotemporal dementia is just one of many conditions—for example, depression, mania, subarachnoid haemorrhage—that can impair decision making. This book is about decisions: how we make them, how they go wrong, and whether it is ethical to improve them through the use of drugs. This may seem like an abstract topic and, admittedly, some of the things we discuss in this book are theoretical and subtle. But subtle is not the same as insignificant.

Decisions are integral to daily life. From picking an entrée to crossing a street to taking a new job and beyond, our actions—and, in a very real sense, our *selves*—are the product of our decisions.

We usually strive to make good ones, but sometimes we make bad ones. As we will see throughout this book, for some people these bad choices are due to identifiable disease processes—in other words: chemical, anatomical, or psychological abnormalities that we can detect and categorize. Wouldn't it be wonderful if scientists and physicians could find an intervention that might alleviate some of the destructive behavioural tendencies seen in these patients? They have. Medications already exist that seem to normalize some of the poor decisions that patients with conditions such as frontotemporal dementia, depression, and mania tend to make. And many more such medications are under development.

The example of our patient in the garden may seem melodramatic, but it is not, and the effects and conditions we describe within this book affect millions of people throughout the world. Patients with these diseases, and many others, lose the fundamental ability to weigh evidence, balance the influence of emotions, and make a decision that advances their best interests. Though its effects can be severe, a decision-making deficit is often difficult to recognize and address, precisely because decision making is complex and we often take it for granted. It is probably fairly easy to recall complex or difficult decisions that we have made: should I go to university; shall I buy this car; would I benefit from investing in a particular company or stock; should I stay married; should I change professions? However, decisions also occur in more mundane ways throughout the day: tie or no tie; walk, drive, or bike; tea or coffee? These latter examples are clearly identifiable decisions, and are usually simpler to make.[1] But 'decision making' applies to more than the making of clear-cut choices. In other words, the cognition of decision making is far more involved and fundamental to our experience.

As we delve more deeply into the topic of decision making, we must keep in mind that nearly everything we do and many things we feel are the result of decisions—even though we often do not think of them as such. For instance, consider this example. You are watching a football match at a pub, and a drunk patron is staggering around and being obnoxious. What do you do? Do you avert your eyes? Do you ask the bartender to eject the patron? Do you shout, 'Sit down'? These actions—or inactions—are manifestations of decisions. More subtly still, what you *feel* may well be the result of a decision. Do you feel irritated? Do you feel threatened? Do you start to feel irritated and then recall your own boorish behaviour during university and decide you have no right to judge? It is impossible to catalogue all of the possible decisions in even the simplest situation, and we do not intend to. We merely want to emphasize how ingrained the decision-making process is to everyday experience, and how the cognition of *decisions* can encompass changes that are not perceptible to anyone else. When we speak of decisions, it is important to remember how much of our experience and identity is connected to these seemingly simple events.

What it means to decide

Let's start with the word *decision*. A *decision* is taken to mean "the making up of one's mind on any point or course of action",[2] usually after examining a question (either consciously or unconsciously). Making up one's mind on a matter is slightly different from forming an opinion on a matter, which in technical terms is considered a judgement. For instance, holding the opinion (judgement) that classic rock is enjoyable is different from deciding to attend a Rolling Stones concert. Although the two—decisions and judgements—are technically different entities, judgements certainly influence decision making, and in practice it can be very difficult to draw a distinct line between the two. Furthermore, the experimental evidence we cite in this book suggests that judgements and decisions both go wrong in similar ways. Thus, for simplicity's sake, we will treat judgements and decisions as similar entities. In this chapter we will largely be concerning ourselves with the processes by which we arrive at our judgements and decisions.

We go through a conscious period of deliberation for only a tiny fraction of decisions; many, if not the majority, are made subconsciously. In actuality, in many cases 'deliberations' are simply the justifications we make up after the fact for decisions that are made instantaneously. We all know this from our own experience; we often think of reasons for our behaviour *post facto*. For example, you may decide to buy a car that is more expensive than another because you prefer the way it looks. However, you may justify this extra expense by convincing yourself that you have bought the more expensive car on the basis of safety features. But any judgement or decision, even a simple one, is the outcome of a complex set of processes.[3] The key processes involved are:

1. the discovery of information;
2. parsing of information and choosing of relevant information;
3. combining this information in a way that may or may not inform an eventual decision;
4. receiving results and learning from outcomes.

In reality, the stages that lead to a decision are not pristinely distinct, nor are they necessarily conscious. Nor do they all necessarily occur at the time you are confronted with the decision—for instance, you may have discovered the relevant information long before. The four-step model of the decision-making process is a simplification that glosses over many other influences, vagaries, and feedback loops, but it can help us understand the essential functions that take place.

First, we must discover information in our environments. In discovering such information, an individual clarifies which environmental cues he considers to be relevant sources of information. Then, once a decision is made, we learn from the feedback that follows it.[4]

Even though this series of steps may not always be as distinct as it is in theory, we can still see each phase at work in a simple thought experiment. For instance, suppose a friend is deciding whether to wear an overcoat. This decision is primarily based on expectations about the temperature for the day. To gather information about the decision, one basic method could be to look out a window to see if it is raining, hailing, snowing, sunny, etc. But perhaps our friend lives in London, and the weather can change quickly, so the current weather conditions are not much of a guide. In order to acquire additional information and hopefully make a more accurate judgement, he turns on the television and flips to the weather channel, or looks at the forecast on the Internet. Once the various bits of information have been acquired, they need to be combined in some way to allow him to arrive at a conclusion about the temperature, which may in turn inform his decision to wear a wool coat or just a T-shirt when he leaves home. However, past experience and feedback can also inform a decision. Perhaps our friend wore a T-shirt last week thinking that it would be warm because it was sunny, but a cold wind sprang up in the afternoon, or perhaps he initially decides to wear a coat this time but is too hot as soon as he steps outside; both of these experiences will influence his judgement and eventual final decision. Perhaps our friend also resents needing to wear warm clothing in, let us say, June, and that emotional state (resentment) influences his decision to purposely wear inappropriately insubstantial clothing.

To go into a bit more detail about the first two of these theoretical steps, research on the processes by which we arrive at our conclusions has shown that over time, people are able to 'pick up' on various aspects of information in an experimental setting [3]. As we might expect, it is difficult to predict how a particular person will gather such information. Some people acquire too much information, while others gather too little information. Only rarely do people acquire the optimal (as mathematically determined) amount of information needed [4, 5], implying that there is perhaps some sort of trade-off between the energy needed to acquire the various bits of information and the accuracy of that judgement. One paper suggested that when we make decisions, we may usually look for solutions that are simply 'good enough' [6], meaning that people are not interested in using all their mental faculties and energy to seek out the optimal amount or type of information. For instance, so long as we are eventually able to join our friends for dinner at a particular restaurant, it may not be worth our effort to research the various available routes and determine the most efficient way to get to the restaurant. All of these qualifications should indicate that the four-step model of decision making begins to break down almost immediately and provides an incomplete picture of a complicated cognitive process. However, 'gathering' and 'parsing' information is necessary to make the decision.

Once the various pieces of information are collected they must be combined, which can be done using any number of strategies. The two most commonly discussed strategies are the weighted (compensatory) and the non-weighted (non-compensatory) strategies.

In a compensatory strategy, people place weighted values on particular characteristics of the decision. For instance, if you are trying to decide which pastry you would prefer to eat, each different characteristic might be weighted differently: perhaps the volume of fruit filling is given a weight of 7 (on a scale from 1 to 10), whereas total sweetness is given a weight of 3, and the number of calories is given a 2. Once the weights are calculated (unconsciously in many cases), then the overall sum of the characteristics for individual puddings may result in your leaning towards the apple turnover rather than the éclair as your preferred option.[5]

A classic example of using weighted pieces of information in order to arrive at a conclusion can be found in medicine. Diagnosticians employ such a strategy to arrive at the *most likely* diagnosis given a set of particular symptoms. Unfortunately, experts' judgements are often inferior when compared with a computer algorithm's judgements about a particular diagnosis after being given the same information (which is not to say that clinicians' judgements are often inaccurate!) [7]. Human beings are susceptible to a host of factors that an algorithm is not, including fatigue, framing (which we will review shortly), and cases with which the doctor has had recent experience.[6] On the flip side, clinicians are better than computers at judging which individual bits of information should be combined in order to arrive at a global judgement, so the computer's apparent diagnostic ability actually depends on sophisticated preliminary work done by a human operator.[7] In addition, it seems that patients generally trust doctors more than they trust a computer's recommendation, so doctors are unlikely to become redundant in the near future [8]. With compensatory decision-making strategies, the value or accuracy of the decision ultimately depends on the subject having sufficient information and understanding the relationships between the various pieces of information that influence a decision.

On the other hand, *non*-compensatory strategies of combining information focus on discriminating one alternative from another, most often by searching for a recognizable feature that differs between them. This strategy is dubbed 'take the best', and relies on recognition of at least one feature so as to avoid guessing. For example, supposing you were asked: *Which University of Cambridge college is older—Pembroke or Selwyn?* If you don't recognize either name—and the majority of people would not—then you will have to guess, and there is a 50 per cent chance that the answer is wrong. If you recognize that Pembroke College is, in fact, one of the 31 Cambridge colleges but you don't recognize the name of Selwyn College, then you may respond that Pembroke is older than Selwyn simply because you recognize Pembroke and choose the alternative that you recognize (the 'best' option). This happens to be the correct answer, but the strategy for arriving at the decision is clearly unreliable. If you happen to be more intimately acquainted with the history of Cambridge and already know that Pembroke was founded in 1347 but Selwyn was not founded until 1882, then you will have answered correctly without relying on a risky strategy. As we can see, non-compensatory decision making relies on the decision maker having sufficient accurate information on which to base the decision. In the absence of such information, or if the information is actually inaccurate, the subject ends up simply guessing. This is more common than we might like to admit: often times we do not have to hand the necessary information for making a decision logically, and then we fall back on strategies that are not logical and will be unreliable.

Weighted and non-weighted strategies are two ways of explaining the influence of gathered information. But the context of any decision goes beyond the gathering or combining of information. For example, a recent study by researchers at Cornell University found that something as simple as being in the same room as a bottle of hand sanitizer was associated with people expressing more conservative social and political opinions [9]. The presence of subconscious disgust—which, in this study, was influenced by environmental reminders of germs and dirtiness—was enough to affect judgements.[8] This is an example of how context can affect decision making independently of the facts involved, and it is absolutely the case that a decision is hardly ever made in isolation from its context. When making a decision there are usually various options that the individual can decide between, and a variety of circumstances such as perceived probability and value that bear on the options.

For instance, imagine that you have just been given a bonus, and you want to spend some of it by taking your partner on a mini-holiday, but now you have to decide just where you want to go: to London or the Italian Amalfi coast. In real life, many circumstances—cost, weather, number of people travelling, etc.—related to each of the options would be relevant, but for the purposes of this example, we will just focus on weather. Then the possible outcomes of the trip are: 1) a rainy holiday in London, 2) a sunny holiday in London, 3) a rainy holiday on the Amalfi coast, or 4) a sunny holiday on the Amalfi coast. Although the true outcome (whether it will rain or not in each of the places during your holiday) is unknown at the time of decision making, we can analyse the probability of each outcome. We can also determine how we think the potential outcomes might affect us.

In theory, it should be possible to choose the option that seems most likely to give the highest value to the decision maker given the probabilities of various circumstances. It may seem very orderly and sensible that each decision is the result of scores of these micro-judgements/decisions. Yet in reality, even this degree of order is an illusion, because people are generally very bad at judging and assigning probabilities in a formal manner.

Because of this, instances of 'probability' factoring into a decision will likely not involve mathematically derived probabilities, but rather a sort of shorthand for *the outcome I think is most likely*. You may have done this a moment ago, when we gave the example of probabilities of rainfall in London versus the Amalfi coast. You may have thought (we did!) that London is far more likely to be rainy, but in fact it is more complicated than that. It rains more often in London, but Naples has about 50 per cent more precipitation per year.[9] So perhaps it would be more accurate to say that you are more likely to get wet in London but more likely to get soaked in Naples. Or perhaps not—other factors such as the season also play a part. As another example of how probabilities can be unexpectedly slippery, consider the following [10]:

> Linda is 31 years old, single, outspoken and very bright. She majored in philosophy. As a student she was deeply concerned with the issues of discrimination and social justice, and also participated in anti-nuclear demonstrations.
>
> Pick a number from 0 (not probable) to 100 (certain) to indicate that Linda is:
> 1. a bank cashier;
> 2. a bank cashier and active in the feminist movement.

In experiments where this question was asked, many people responded that option two was more probable, by giving it a higher number.

However, it is impossible for option two, which is a subset of the first option, to be more probable; everyone who belongs to the category described in option two also belongs to the category described in option one (see Figure 1). Those who choose option two are not actually answering the question *Which is more probable?* but rather, *Which is more congruent?* Erroneous assumptions of this type often lead people astray and prevent them from properly weighing the laws of probability.[10]

So we have seen that, in practice, judging probabilities of various potential outcomes is actually a very subjective and imprecise activity. The same is true when assigning a value to the potential outcome of a decision. Even in cases where the value can be quantified, different people will respond differently, as will the same person in different circumstances. For instance, £50 probably has a greater value to a poor graduate student than it does to a multimillionaire, and a free meal is valued more when one is hungry than when one is full. Moreover, preferences and what people value can reverse within a matter of minutes—as anyone who has gone food shopping while hungry can attest. The orderly four-step decision-making process we described above is, at best, an approximation, and glosses over some very sophisticated and subtle cognitive functions that are not yet well understood. However, this model does describe how we gather, process and re-evaluate the evidence that informs our decisions at more of a macro level.

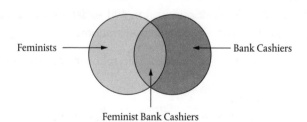

FIGURE 1 Venn diagram of feminists and cashiers showing that the proportion of feminist cashiers must be smaller than the proportion of cashiers in a given population.

We should conclude by stressing that these subjectivities are not defects, deficiencies, or pathologies. They are not the sort of deficient or abnormal decision making that would be treated by the methods discussed in Chapter 4. On the contrary, they are part of the normal decision-making process, because any number of extraneous factors normally enter into our decisions. The basic question that still remains is: *What influences external to the four-step decision process can sway the choice between various courses of action?* We have hinted at these in a general way (mood, probability, value, etc.), but the remainder of this chapter will address some specific factors—framing, risk aversion, time, and emotions—in more detail, and look at evidence for how they are able to influence decisions. You can think of these additional factors as coming into play in step three of the decision-making model (combining information). These factors do not necessarily affect what information you notice, or what information you think is relevant. Instead, they have a huge, and measurable, impact on how we synthesize information and eventually make decisions based upon it. These factors are also integral to the decision-making disorders and treatments we will discuss later.

Framing: it's not what you said, it's how you said it

Framing refers to *how* the information that will be used to make a decision is presented, and it is incredibly influential on how that information is processed and employed. For instance, when trying to make a decision between two different treatments for lung cancer, the treatment a patient chooses may reflect whether the information was presented as the number of people who *die* from each treatment versus the number who *survive* each treatment. In this example, the following two scenarios are statistically equivalent, but framed very differently:

1. Of 100 people having surgery, on average, 10 will die in treatment, 32 will have died by one year and 66 will have

died by five years. Of 100 people having radiation therapy, on average, none will die during treatment, 23 will die by one year, and 78 will die by five years.

2. Of 100 people having surgery, on average, 90 will survive the treatment, 68 will survive for one year and 34 will survive for five years. Of 100 people having radiation therapy, on average, all will survive the treatment, 77 will survive for one year, and 22 will survive for five years.

In this example, surgery carries a greater chance of death during treatment, but also a greater chance that the patient will survive to five years. However, studies have found that patients are more likely to opt for radiation therapy than surgery in scenario 1 (the negative framing), but more likely to opt for surgery when the framing was that of scenario 2 (the positive framing) [11]. Surgery is often a high-risk, high-reward proposition; emphasizing the positive (reward) aspect makes people more accepting of the risks, even when the risk is death. The presentation of the information is incredibly powerful, and it is apparent how this knowledge can be used to direct decisions in particular ways.

Medical treatments are one notable area where framing plays a huge role in influencing outcomes, though in general the people involved do not have a specific agenda. The situation is very different in other contexts such as politics and political polling, where wording can produce seemingly huge swings of opinion on a given topic.

Because framing has the ability to alter the public's perception, politicians choose their words carefully in posing and answering questions, and many even employ experts to help them determine the best way to phrase something. Frank Luntz is a famous political pollster and strategist who has worked mainly with conservative parties in the USA and the UK.[11] He is known for 'testing language' and finding the particular manner in which to communicate an idea in a way that might sway opinion [12]. He famously coined the phrase

'Death Tax' rather than 'Inheritance Tax'. He includes his reasoning for using 'Death Tax' in the appendix of a memo sent to Republicans, fondly entitled 'The 14 Words Never to Use' [13]. He writes that, 'While a sizeable 68 per cent of America thinks the Inheritance/Estate Tax is unfair, *fully 78 per cent think that the Death Tax is unfair*',[12] and 'an over-whelming majority [of sampled individuals] would repeal the death tax'. He recommends to Republicans that, 'If you want to kill the estate tax, call it a death tax'. In the same memo, he advises the smart Republican to avoid phrases such as 'drilling for oil', 'foreign trade', 'globalization', as well as criticizing the 'government' (since the local governments are responsible for cleaning up streets, providing police and transport services). Instead, he advocates 'exploring for energy', 'international trade', 'free market economy', and criticizing 'Washington' (which he suggests has the connotation of a bureaucratic, red-tape-ridden epicentre of taxes and regulations). His suggestions have proven influential and contributed to winning campaigns.

While we should be aware of the immense importance of framing, it is also important to remember that framing is not necessarily a conscious biasing or misdirection (though it can be). We should all be slightly sceptical when presented with the results of any one poll, but that does not mean the pollsters necessarily did anything wrong. The ambiguity and subtlety of wording items such as poll questions or ballot initiatives may simply be the result of writers trying to engage more effectively with the human decision-making process... and framing is just one of several factors that can influence it greatly.

Risk aversion: please don't hurt me

Risk aversion and risk seeking are also important factors in why peo-ple make the decisions that they do [14]. Risk aversion means that people will tend to take a guaranteed gain if one is available (even if for a small reward), rather than risk losing. This phenomenon holds true even in cases in which the subject stands to win a larger amount.

For example, risk aversion means that, on average, a subject will take a guaranteed payout of £5, rather than flipping a coin with the chance of winning or losing £10 riding on the outcome.

On the other hand, in a situation in which they are guaranteed to lose something, people seem more willing to gamble and risk losing a larger amount. In other words, faced with a choice between taking a guaranteed loss of £200 or doing a double-or-nothing coin flip, many people will choose the coin flip. This is called risk-seeking behaviour. These phenomena are easy to quantify with cash values, but of course they also apply to more abstract types of gain or loss. It has also been shown that people prefer to remain in a known and familiar status quo situation rather than risk moving to a new condition that is unknown and unfamiliar (and perhaps reflects a more uncertain future) [15]. This phenomenon is known as 'status quo bias' and is a major factor in real-world decisions that involve potential change, such as deciding whether to switch careers, or even to get a new hairstyle.

Time…to make a decision

Since most decisions are made very quickly and subconsciously, time may not at first appear to be a major factor in the majority of them. However, time can be a very powerful influence in at least two ways.

The first way has to do with the temporal disconnect involved in many decisions, i.e. you have to make a decision in the present, but the outcome will often not be known until well into the future. This can play an important role in cases of immediate versus delayed gratification—do you choose to have the reward now, or do you choose to wait until some point in the future when the reward may be different? We have all had to decide between immediate gratification and delayed gratification at some point in our lives—dessert versus dieting is perhaps the most clear-cut example—but this phenomenon is not always so benign.

Addiction is perhaps one of the more infamous instances of an inability to delay gratification. Studies of activity in the brain using the technique of functional magnetic resonance imaging (fMRI)[13] have shown that immediate and delayed outcomes activate different parts of the brain, and can also be correlated with the amount of brain activity within those regions [16, 17]. People can usually control the desire for immediate gratification by specifically focusing on the reasons for delaying or avoiding the particular temptation at hand, but once distracted from those reasons, it is much easier, and more common, to choose the immediate reward [18].

Time is also a factor when decisions must be made under perceived or actual time pressure, e.g. you must make a decision *now*, otherwise you might miss out on an opportunity. This is another powerful, yet subtle, effect. Different people react in different ways; for instance, for some individuals, status quo bias is activated when they feel they are being pushed too hard or too far. These people simply shut down under pressure and refuse to make a decision that would result in change from the status quo. However, this is not the only, or even the most common, reaction to pressure, which is one reason why sales agents are keen to remind you that you might miss out on a great opportunity if you do not act now. The results can be seen in many everyday examples: purchases that we wish could be returned (perhaps that vacation timeshare you were talked into?), and big life decisions that we wish we could take back (for instance, the mayfly-like marriages coming out of Las Vegas).

Although there is considerable variation between different people, in general it is much more difficult to make an accurate decision under time pressure. As a result, a large part of the training for professions that involve making important time-sensitive decisions (for instance, doctors or military personnel) is dedicated to reducing this pressure. These individuals replicate high-pressure situations as much as possible beforehand, so that as much of the activity as possible is second nature, without requiring new decisions to be made.

That way, when the truly unexpected occurs and must be addressed *now*, they are in a better position than most people to assess the legitimately important information, and free to use the time available to make the best possible decision under the circumstances.

Another benefit of this type of repetitive high-pressure training is to ameliorate the unpleasant emotions that usually accompany stress or pressure. For instance, Tom Wolfe memorably described the process of training early astronauts as primarily being one of desensitization, of making the stresses of spaceflight "as familiar, as routine, as workaday as an office" and thereby "enabling one to think and use his hands normally in a novel environment" [19].[14] This approach to training gives us a hint of the last important decision making factor we will discuss at present: emotions.

Emotions: I feel good (or not)

As we will discuss in more detail in future chapters, emotions are an important factor that influences our decisions. Decisions do not occur in an emotional vacuum. This will be familiar to most of us; we know instinctively that we will make different choices if we are happy or sad, excited or wary, etc. Emotions play a huge role in shaping decision making, but they are sometimes downplayed or ignored precisely because they are so common, and usually subtle.

Antonio Damasio and his colleagues have proposed one of the most influential theories of how emotions affect decision making. This collection of ideas is referred to as the Somatic Marker Hypothesis [20]. According to this theory, there is a mechanism for learning to discriminate good responses from bad responses, and it likely employs certain structures in the prefrontal cortex. This system allows an individual to associate patterns of activity in the body's systems (called somatic states) with particular stimuli. For example, choosing to go to the gym may lead to trepidation, physical discomfort, an endorphin rush, satisfaction, etc. This state, or cluster of states, is then labelled (for lack of a better term), stored in our memory systems, and recalled the next time we are deciding whether or not to go to the gym. A somatic state can be reactivated by a similar stimulus in the future, so that an individual's decision-making processes are affected by the prior labelling of the somatic state and outcome as good or bad. There are other theories about how emotions arise and ultimately impact cognition; we mention this theory only to emphasize how complicated and subtle the role of emotions actually is. Although the mechanisms of emotions deserve further research, we are primarily concerned with the effect of emotions—and here we are on more solid ground.

Certainly, emotions have caused many individuals to lean towards or away from some decision at some point in their lives, and they can even seem to short-circuit or bypass the entire decision-making process we described above. This is particularly true of 'snap decisions'. In other cases our emotional state can seem to be the primary factor in the decision. Even after we have gathered the evidence and made a pro and con list, in the end the final decision may rest on which option a person simply *prefers*—the one that makes him or her happier, or relieves a particular emotional pressure. Indeed, even if a pro/con list might indicate that you should make a particular decision based on the value you have given various components of decision, you might keep fiddling with the weights on the criteria until the outcome indicated is the one you desired in the first place. Emotions are an aspect of decision making that cannot be ignored, and yet the research community has only recently begun to display widespread interest in the emotional component of decision making.

It was in 1980 that a social psychologist named Robert Zajonc drew attention to the fact that emotional reactions—liking the creaminess of ice cream, disliking mouldy cheese, preferring cats to dogs—are not necessarily post-cognitive processes (in other words, a person does not need to have knowledge or to have processed information about the item before forming an opinion).

He also pointed out that cognitive psychologists in his day simply ignored emotional states. But as Zajonc noted:

> Most of the time, information collected about alternatives serves us less for making a decision than for justifying it afterwards…We buy the cards we 'like', choose the jobs and houses that we find 'attractive', and then justify those choices by various reasons that might appear convincing to others…We need not convince ourselves. *We* know what we like [21].[15]

Zajonc's discussions about thinking and feeling focus on 'hot' decisions in particular. 'Hot' decisions are those that involve an emotional component, and are distinct from purely rational, 'cold' decisions.

These concepts of 'hot' and 'cold' decisions are central to the rest of this book, so they are worth exploring in some detail. 'Cold' decisions are thought not to have an emotional or risk component [22]. These are decisions such as which grocery items you need to buy in order to make a particular meal for supper, and they are about as straightforward as human decisions can be; though, as we will see later, this is not the same as saying the process never breaks down. 'Hot' decisions, on the other hand, have an emotional component or may involve weighing rewards and punishments [22]. For example, the decision whether to continue dating your current partner or accept a date with someone you recently met and you are very attracted to is a hot decision—surely you cannot get away from emotions in that situation, even if you try to be rational. Decisions made under extreme emotional stress—everything from quitting a job to committing a crime *in the heat of the moment*—are also hot decisions.[16]

Some of the links between emotions and decisions will be obvious from personal experience or popular culture. For instance, researchers from Massachusetts Institute of Technology and Carnegie Mellon revealed that males who were in a state of sexual arousal described themselves as being more willing to engage in morally questionable behaviour and more willing to have unsafe sex [23]. Few of us will be surprised by these results. But the effects of emotion are not always so intuitively clear. Other researchers have found that when people are asked to imagine being in a good or a bad mood, they are more likely to choose to watch a comedy than if their attention is not drawn to mood at all. In other words, it is possible to influence the decision-making process and make people more likely to choose differently merely by bringing attention to mood [24]. And oddest of all, consciously putting yourself in a certain emotional state can affect the decisions you make later—in other words, an emotion that we deliberately elicit can be just as real, or influential, as an emotion that arises from an experience. This is the basis of behavioural therapy for mood disorders such as depression. Therapy encourages patients to cultivate a certain mood in order to make it more likely that they will choose behaviours that reinforce that mood.

This is all by way of saying that although emotions definitely have an effect on decision making, we are far from truly understanding how that influence operates. Nevertheless, the connections between emotions and decisions can sometimes be illuminated by studying cases where both are impaired. For example, many people suffer from pathologies that leave them struggling to make good decisions, and all too often the mechanism seems to be an illness that affects their mood (e.g. depression). Since we know that mood and emotions affect decision making, it is unsurprising that individuals with mood or emotional disorders often suffer from impaired decision making as well. How do we know about these pathologies? What effects do they have on the brain? Our next chapter will address these questions and pave the way for an examination of risky behaviour and the medications that can alleviate it.

2

PEERING INSIDE
THE 'BLACK BOX'

In all science, error precedes the truth, and it is better it should go first than last.   Sir Hugh Walpole, novelist

Oh, how far we've come

For much of man's history, we have not understood the brain. Four millennia ago, when preparing bodies for the afterlife, Egyptians used to remove and discard the brain as worthless, while taking great care to preserve the heart, stomach, liver, and other organs. A look back at the history of investigations into the brain is a humbling reminder of how far we have come in understanding our own minds, and also how far we still have to go.

For thousands of years, people speculated about the relationship between personality traits and specific organs,[1] but it was not until the late 18th and early 19th centuries that the brain was suggested to be the seat of mental activity.[2] In 1819, Franz Gall attempted to relate an individual's personal characteristics and skull shape in a scientific manner. This was the beginning of phrenology, the belief that certain brain areas have specific innate functions (or faculties), and that these functions are related to the shape, lumps, and bumps of the skull (see Figure 2).[3]

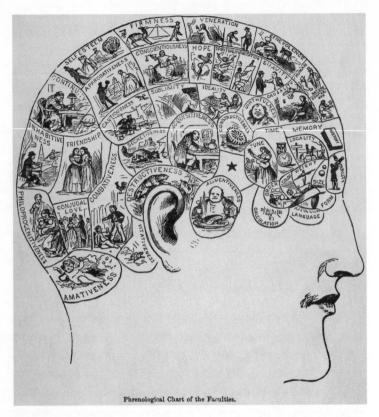

Phrenological Chart of the Faculties.

FIGURE 2 A phrenological chart from the 19th century showing areas described by Gall. Certain areas of the skull were supposedly related to characteristics such as self-esteem, tune, conjugal love, and destructiveness, among others.

© Bettmann/CORBIS

Phrenology was taken quite seriously by some, including British prime minister Lloyd George and countless other people interested in hiring a new employee,[4] knowing their children's futures, or finding a suitable spouse. Others saw it as good-humoured fun,[5] and still others used it to support racist beliefs.[6] Although phrenology has long been out of favour in the scientific community, it can still be seen in various popular culture media, usually with individuals poking fun.[7] Some have argued that phrenology was the beginning of modern neuroscientific methodology, even though phrenology has since been discredited. However, phrenology's suggestion that mental processes can be localized to the brain has paved the way for methods of interpreting the brain's organization,[8] theories of psychology and imaging, and modern neuroscience.

Still, however, phrenology was focused on the skull...not the brain. Many early 19th-century scientists suspected that the frontal area of the brain—the area of the brain we largely concern ourselves with in this book—did not have any specific function. However, in the mid 19th century, the (scientifically) fortuitous, unrepeated happenstance of Phineas Gage's accident—which involved an iron rod, some gunpowder, a horrific head wound, and changed behaviour—shed some unexpected light on the functionality of the frontal brain (see Figure 3). Thereafter, some researchers sought to expand their explorations of the brain, though not always with benign results.

The shift to a brain-centric focus for research was by no means swift or universal. Nearly a century after Gage's accident had suggested a link between specific brain functions and specific brain areas, the psychological movement known as Behaviourism was still hugely influential. Behaviourists focused primarily on what are known as learned behaviours and conditioned responses. They were unable to test what occurred within the 'black box' of the brain, so they focused instead on measurable inputs and observable behaviours that were independent of conscious experience or 'the mind'. Behaviourists presumed that only external changes could be reliably examined. If we asked a Behaviourist how best to study a human being, he would respond with something like: Put him in a situation and observe whether his behaviour changes or remains static, and if his behaviour changes, how it changes.[9] By contrast, contemporary cognitive researchers are more interested in what lies beneath the veneer of

(A)

(B)

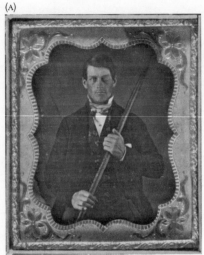

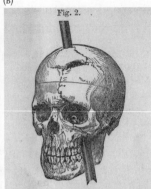

Front and lateral view of the cranium, representing the direction in which the iron traversed its cavity; the present appearance of the line of fracture, and also the large anterior fragment of the frontal bone, which was entirely detached, replaced, and partially re-united.

FIGURE 3 (A) In July 2009, discovery of a daguerreotype portrait of brain-injury survivor Phineas Gage was announced. The daguerreotype shows Mr Gage holding the tamping iron that injured him. (B) View of the skull showing the course that the rod took through Mr Gage's head.

(A) From the collection of Jack and Beverly Wilgus; (B) Publications of the Massachusetts Medical Society (v. 2 (1868): 327–347).

behaviour, and it is widely felt that the field of cognitive studies grew in part as a reaction *against* the methodologies and theories proposed by Behaviourists.[10]

Cognitive neuroscience and cognitive psychology focus on what Behaviorism neglected: the biological origins of human thought and cognition.[11] Additionally, the cognitive fields approach questions of the mind using scientific methodology—formulation of hypotheses, design of experiments, and data collection. Contemporary neuroscience research is in some ways a complex edifice built on the most random foundations, a discipline where even the most modern work is shaped by a fascinating history of errors and discoveries. This raises an obvious question: how does one construct objective ways in which to peer into the brain; how does one attempt to see what is in the 'black box'?

Learning from nature's accidents
(and human manipulation)

The most basic division in the brain is between the right and left hemispheres.[12] You may even have heard someone describe himself/herself as a 'right brain' or 'left brain' person. These terms have entered into popular usage because of studies that have differentiated the functionality of the two halves. The left half of the brain is—to use very general terms—the logical, calculating, language-based half; the right side, on the other hand, tends to function in more creative and artistic ways, dealing with 'gestalts'.[13]

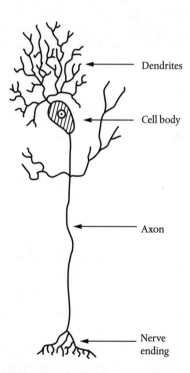

Dendrites

Cell body

Axon

Nerve ending

FIGURE 4 Basic diagram of a neuron, which is one type of cell in the brain. Electrical activity travels from the dendrites along the axon towards the nerve ending.

Although incomplete, one method of understanding the role of different parts of the brain is to see what happens to a person's abilities when a particular part of the brain is damaged. Cognitive scientists and clinicians can study people who have unfortunately suffered from traumatic incidents (such as was the case with Phineas Gage), strokes, and also those with abnormal brain anatomy or traumatic events at birth. When such events occur, researchers can study the resulting changes in cognitive function and correlate these changes with the structures that are damaged or absent.

For example, consider the unfortunate history of frontal lobotomies. In 1949, António Caetano de Abreu Freire Egas Moniz won the Nobel Prize in Medicine for standardizing the practice of trauma to the frontal brain. Dr Egas Moniz had developed the leucotomy, which was adapted by Dr Walter Freeman into the standard lobotomy known today and memorably depicted in the book and film *One Flew Over the Cuckoo's Nest*. To put it plainly, during a lobotomy a surgical tool was inserted through the thin bones of the skull and into the brain, where it was moved around in order to damage connections.[14] This psychosurgery differed from the four-millennia-old Egyptian procedure only in the design of the instrument and a disagreement about how much of the brain was undesirable. Although the lobotomy is no longer used in most countries, it is a stark reminder of the intersection between brain anatomy, interventional methods, and quite dramatic effects on specific aspects of cognitive function.

The frontal lobotomy was a crude intervention, and was used most frequently in the asylum population because it was thought by some to be a cure for the mentally ill (particularly for patients with schizophrenia, since no pharmacological treatment was available at the time). In this narrow sense, it was 'effective': patients who underwent 'treatment' were more docile and less likely to harm themselves, while still being able to perform basic functions such as feeding themselves. But lobotomies were also noted to dehumanize the patients, resulting in vacant stares and an inability to rouse an emotional reaction.[15] Howard Dully was a 12-year-old boy when he was lobotomized, and his brother's description of him after the fact was as follows:

> You were sitting up in the bed, with two black eyes...you looked listless. And sad. Like a zombie. It's not a nice word to use, but it's the only word to use. You were zoned out and staring. I was in shock. And sad. It was just terribly sad. [25][16]

Unfortunately, the procedure was quite prevalent. It was significantly cheaper in the mid 1900s to lobotomize an individual (approximately $200) than to keep him incarcerated or in an asylum (thousands of dollars). Upwards of 40,000 lobotomies were performed in the United States, and nearly 20,000 were performed in Great Britain.

In 1977, the US National Committee for the Protection of Human Subjects of Biomedical and Behavioral Research completed an investigation into the benefits of the frontal lobotomy and ruled that this form of surgery, when extremely limited and properly performed, could have positive effects. However, there was a fair amount of disagreement as to how effective the procedure was,[17] and by this time pharmacological therapies had become more available and the lobotomy had already fallen into disuse. Frontal lobotomies were banned in most states in the USA, and in most countries around the world in the 1970s.

The sad case of lobotomies is one reason why modern researchers are confident about the role that the frontal lobe plays in emotion and executive or complex cognitive functioning. It is also a powerful warning about the ethics of permanent interventions and of the difficulty of targeting specific surgical sites in the brain.[18]

Other accidents—traumatic, vascular (e.g. stroke), surgical—have shed some light on the functions of other brain areas. For instance, an area of the brain known as Broca's area is involved in speech production.[19] Individuals who have damage to this area can understand what is said to them and follow commands, but cannot readily communicate because their language production is affected. On the other hand, individuals with damage to Wernicke's area have difficulty comprehending speech.[20] They cannot follow commands. The speech production that remains is fluent with a relatively normal cadence and syntax, but completely unintelligible.

Anatomical methods are a crude way to understand brain function, because an absent or abnormal structure may not exactly correlate with the change in behaviour. Grey matter (cell bodies) and white matter (axons that carry information along pathways) are often both located within a given region; if a particular area of the brain is abnormal, it is difficult to know whether behavioural changes are due to damage to the cells or the pathways coursing through the area. However, though crude, this method of anatomical correlation can begin to reveal something about the function of different areas of the brain.

Structure, not function

Throughout much of neuroscientific history, changes in symptoms were the diagnostic tool by which brain lesions were localized, and usually the presumed lesions were confirmed at the time of autopsy. However, now we can correlate patients' symptoms with distinctive anatomical features, as well as visualize changes to the brain's anatomical structure by using various imaging technologies, such as computerized tomography (CT) and magnetic resonance imaging (MRI). This ability has clinical and research benefits because the affected area can be more reliably identified, and problems can be seen *in vivo* rather than pieced together over years from examining autopsy reports and correlating them with reports of patient symptoms. In cases of suspected anatomical disturbance, CT and MRI scans can be used to determine structural abnormalities, while positron emission tomography (PET) and functional MRI (fMRI) can be used to investigate brain function. We shall address these types of imaging technology in turn.

CT scans provide structural information. They do this by taking a series of X-rays of the head in many different directions (the machine rotates while the patient remains stationary). Once a computer program determines—using various mathematical calculations—how much of an X-ray beam is absorbed by the brain, a 2D image can be produced to reflect the composition of the brain tissue (see Figure 5). The head is composed of many different substances, including bone, air, blood, water, and neurons, but in general, as the density of a tissue increases, so does its whiteness on a CT scan. The scanner builds up a complete image from multiple smaller slices, and there are now programs that convert 2D images into 3D brain reconstructions. In order to better understand how image reconstruction works, imagine that you have separate 2D images that show the layout of each floor of a building. By combining these images in a computer, you can generate a 3D model that more clearly shows features that span different floors—such as stairs or multistorey atriums. CT image reconstruction functions in an analogous manner.

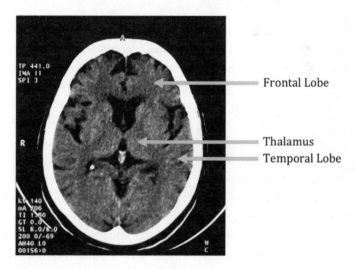

FIGURE 5 A normal CT scan of the head showing a portion of the frontal and temporal lobes, as well as bilateral thalami. Brain tissue is grey, whereas bone is white.

© xpixel/Shutterstock.com

MRI scans also provide anatomical information, but do so using a different principle from CT, and without exposing a patient to radiation. The subject is instructed to lie still on his back in a non-metal tube and a cylindrical supercooled[21] magnet around the tube creates a large, stable magnetic field, which alters the alignment of hydrogen nuclei in the patient's body. A pulsed radio frequency field then causes these hydrogen nuclei to emit characteristic radio energy of their own.[22] A sensor can read these frequencies and use them to construct an image that shows the different kinds of tissue in a particular part of the body (see Figure 6).

Even though these modes of imaging provide merely structural information, much can still be gleaned from them. For instance, a review of the available literature reveals that depression is associated

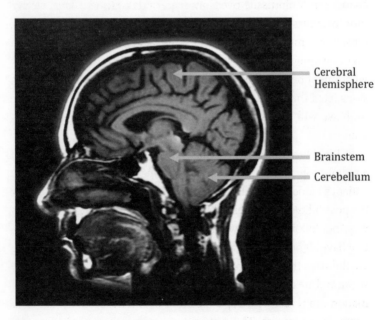

Cerebral
Hemisphere

Brainstem
Cerebellum

FIGURE 6 An MRI scan showing detail of the midsagittal brain, including the cerebral hemisphere, cerebellum, and brainstem.

Courtesy of OUP Picturebank/Photodisc

with consistent structural MRI findings such as decreased brain volume in distinct parts of the limbic system and orbitofrontal cortex [26]. We will discuss these areas of the brain in more detail in future chapters. Moreover, it seems that this decrease in tissue volume correlates with severity of depression—having the illness for a longer time, having multiple bouts of depression, etc. Thus, structural imaging can provide clues about where researchers might focus further attention, and can also imply a brain basis for disease.

Function, not structure

The above methods of scanning can provide a snapshot of what the brain looks like at a given moment, and can be correlated to show changes in brain tissue over longer periods of time—days, weeks, months, years—but they cannot give any information about brain *activity* on a moment-to-moment basis. If a researcher wants to use brain imaging tools to look into the 'black box' and speculate about what might be going on during specific behaviours, thoughts, decisions, etc., then he must rely on different tools. The first of these tools we will look at is the positron emission tomography (PET) scan.

PET is able to detect the pairs of gamma rays that are emitted when a radioisotope decays.[23] These radioisotopes are introduced into the patient's blood, attached to particular molecules (usually a sugar, but the possibilities are endless[24]). When the isotopes are attached in this way, they follow blood flow, and a scanner can detect areas of the body that have higher concentrations of these particular molecules—these are the areas that are demanding more blood flow, using more blood sugar, and are therefore (presumably) more active. As such, this information can reveal which specific areas within the brain are active at particular moments. The patterns of gamma ray emission can be tracked over time, and changes in those patterns can be correlated with changes in behaviour (see Figure 7). When PET is used with CT or

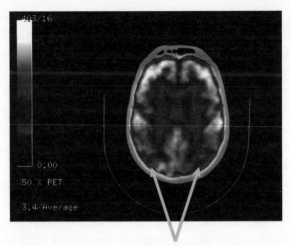

Parietal Lobes

FIGURE 7 PET scan showing relatively decreased activity in both parietal lobes (indicated by the arrows), which is consistent with Alzheimer's disease.
Image Courtesy of Dr Josh Klein.

MRI scans, a researcher can look at a specific anatomical structure and determine whether it is active during a particular process.

Or at least that is the ideal. PET scanning is a powerful tool, particularly in understanding the actions of drugs in the brain. However, like any tool, PET has some limitations, and its particular weaknesses make it more appropriate for measuring metabolic rates (such as in cancer cells) than brain activity. First, building up an image of an active area requires a sustained increase in the amount of gamma radiation emitted. Therefore, the changes seen in activity levels are not temporally precise; in other words, we may know where the changes are taking place, but not how quickly they occur. Second, because image reconstruction relies on coincident (simultaneous) recording of gamma photons, random coincidences can lead to spurious data. Third, the detectors themselves have a refractory period—after one detects a gamma ray, there is a short period in which it cannot detect another. Last, the gamma rays pass through some tissues more easily than others, meaning that the deeper a ray's journey begins, the less likely it is to reach the surface and be detected; so structures deeper in the body automatically have a lower reported number of coincident rays, leading to a lower level of radioactivity on the resulting map. However, there are mathematical algorithms designed to take these limitations into consideration when reconstructing the image, and these maps have proven useful to many different clinical and research professionals.

Similar to PET scanning, functional magnetic resonance imaging (fMRI) also allows researchers a window into the brain. Unlike PET scanning, fMRI is able to do this in a much more spatially precise manner. It does this by directly measuring the haemodynamic (blood) response to neural activity, rather than radioactive decay of metabolic molecules carried in the blood to active brain areas (as in PET).

It has been known since the 1890s that blood and oxygen levels correlate with neuron activity, because active neurons consume oxygen, which is carried in the blood. As a result, it makes sense to state that blood flow increases to areas of the brain that are involved in performing a particular task. Blood flow begins to increase no more than one second after neural activity begins.[25] When oxygenated blood flow increases to a brain region, the local ratio of oxygenated to deoxygenated blood changes. This change in ratio is precisely what is being measured by fMRI, made possible because of Linus Pauling's serendipitous discovery that oxygenated and deoxygenated blood have different magnetic properties. When an individual is placed in an fMRI machine, it is possible to watch the blood-oxygen-level-dependent (BOLD) signal in various brain areas change as the ratio of oxygenated to deoxygenated blood changes.[26] Multiple images are taken and averaged together in order to create a map of activity during a specific task (see Figure 8), and responses to stimuli as close together as one to two seconds can be differentiated. The variety of tasks used is unbelievable, ranging from moving a joystick and

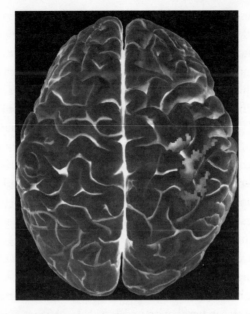

FIGURE 8 The right hemisphere of the brain controls movement on the left side of the body. In this fMRI image, we see that some areas within the right half of the brain become active when the patient's left hand moves. For orientation purposes, the front of the brain is at the top of the image.

© Science Photo Library

individual parts of your body, to looking at images, listening to particular sounds, making gambling decisions, and even being sexually aroused. So PET and fMRI offer methods for determining the location of brain activity, though with some limitations regarding their temporal precision and response time. The shortfalls of fMRI and PET can be addressed to a certain extent by coupling these techniques with the strengths of electroencephalography (EEG) and magnetoencephalography (MEG). EEG and MEG are temporally accurate (on the order of milliseconds) but spatially inaccurate methods that record, respectively, the electrical or magnetic fluctuations of active populations of neurons in the brain.

Some researchers have challenged the relevance of anatomical findings from fMRI and PET studies, saying that these are simply technologically advanced phrenology, providing us with an answer to *Where in the brain?* but not *How?* Anatomical activity findings also do not reveal the ways in which areas work together in order to accomplish a task, only that one or more areas have changes in activity during a task. For instance, a group of scientists recently wrote, quite rightly, that "brain regions are typically engaged by many mental states, and thus a one-to-one mapping between a brain region and a mental state is not possible" [27].

However, advances in mathematical techniques and the use of combinations of the above research modalities have allowed researchers to analyse the connections between brain regions during activity. These observations lead to conclusions that go far beyond the simple correspondence of brain region and particular function. We are starting to be able to link patterns of brain behaviour to specific thoughts and decisions. Thus, by analysing patterns of activation, some researchers have even been able to predict a choice before the subject makes it. This is particularly important in the context of non-invasive brain–machine interfaces. The neuroscientist John-Dylan Haynes suggests that by learning to identify brain activity patterns it is possible to infer what a person is thinking [28]. Brain–machine interfaces are used to help develop techniques that allow individuals to control devices using only their thoughts. These are the techniques that may allow an amputee to control a prosthetic limb, a mute to spell a word, a tetraplegic to steer a wheelchair, or even a monkey to explore his environment without moving [29].

fMRI and PET provide only one type of evidence in our attempts to understand brain function; the data that they provide are combined with data accumulated from other studies. As an analogy, citing one area of the brain as being responsible for, say, reading, is like saying one cylinder of a car engine is responsible for the motion of the car— it is necessary, but the overall state of motion is dependent on a lot of other parts working together in an organized and effective manner.

In science, most advances occur when multiple studies using different techniques imply a harmonious answer. fMRI and PET provide useful data about brain activity that can be correlated with other research paradigms such as neuropsychological testing and the lesion studies mentioned above to expand our understanding. A few words on these neuropsychological testing approaches are appropriate here.

Pen, paper, and PCs

Questionnaires and computer tasks are still the most common neuropsychological testing methods, and they provide researchers with a surprising array of options for testing people.

Computer tasks provide objective information about an individual's performance: reaction times, number of attempts made, correct responses, etc. The variety of computer tasks is essentially limitless; to test different cognitive functions, we could develop a computer task that requires people to remember which six patterns are in which six boxes, a task that requires people to stop themselves from doing something (e.g. pressing a button) when they hear a beep, or a task that asks people to classify facial expressions as happy or sad. In fact, all of these computer tasks exist, and there are many others. These tasks can be done while people are being imaged using fMRI or PET, thus allowing brain localization of regions involved in memory processes, impulse control, emotional recognition, and decision making. Performance can further be correlated with activity or lack of activity in particular regions of the brain. These tasks can be given to both healthy volunteers and patients with mental illness or neurological disorders. For example, the Cambridge Neuropsychological Test Automated Battery (CANTAB) is a collection of computerized neuropsychological tests developed in Cambridge and used throughout the world.[27] CANTABmobile on iPad allows for rapid, easy assessment of cognition and for the screening of memory problems in the elderly for early detection of Alzheimer's disease.

Questionnaires with scales provide a slightly different approach to quantifying brain activity: subjects answer questions such as how impulsive do you consider yourself on a scale from 1 to 10, or how often do you make decisions 'on the fly', with 1 meaning 'never' and 5 meaning 'always'? There are standardized questionnaires (for example, the Barratt Scale of Impulsivity), as well as ones that are designed for a particular study's needs and validated before use in the study. The emotional scales and criteria derived from these data (which we will discuss more in Chapter 3) are an attempt to standardize a very subjective set of experiences and allow objective comparisons between data collected from different people. Questionnaires are often used together with other testing paradigms, such as computer tasks.

Where does all this get us?

As an example of how testing modalities can be used together to collect information about a complex cognitive process, we turn to hot and cold decisions. As discussed in the previous chapter, cold decisions are thought not to have an emotional component and do not involve a risk component—for example, what ingredients do I need to purchase in order to make a certain dish for supper? Hot decisions, on the other hand, have an emotional component or may involve weighing rewards and punishments and assessing risk—for example, should I dump my current partner and call that person I hit it off with last week?

From a scientific point of view, how might one investigate these two types of decisions?[28] One way to model a cold decision is to make a game that requires a decision by the participant without rewarding or punishing that decision. One such computerized game is loosely related to the classic Tower of Hanoi game,[29] and is called the CANTAB Stockings of Cambridge.[30] In this game, participants are asked to move coloured balls on a screen to make an arrangement look like a target arrangement in a specified number of moves (see Figure 9). Using fMRI, researchers have discovered that when healthy people

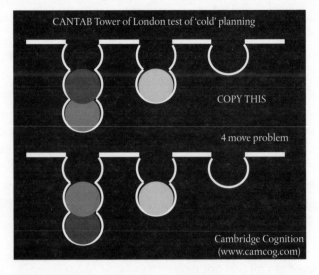

FIGURE 9 CANTAB Stockings of Cambridge computer task (www.camcog .com). The goal of the task is to make the bottom arrangement look like the top arrangement in a specified number of moves of the balls hanging in the pockets (or 'stockings'). This example shows a four-move task.

are performing this task, blood flow increases to a part of their brain known as the dorsolateral ('on the top and to the side') prefrontal cortex (see Figure 10) [30]. People who have damage to this part of their brain also make more errors during the course of the task [31], implying that this brain region is critical for non-emotional decision making.

In a similar way, but by using a very different task, researchers have determined that one area involved in making emotionally laden, hot decisions is the orbitofrontal cortex (the part of the frontal brain above the eye sockets) [32]. This region has increased blood flow during a hot task very different from the Stockings of Cambridge. In fact, patients with dorsolateral prefrontal cortex damage—the same patients who have trouble with the cold decision-making task—can perform this hot task perfectly well.

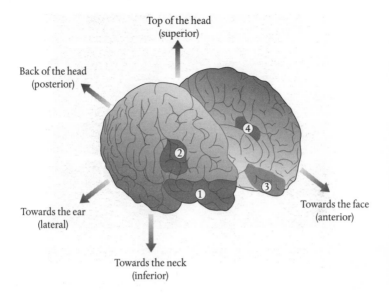

FIGURE 10 Anatomy of the prefrontal cortex, showing (1) orbitofrontal cortex, (2) dorsolateral prefrontal cortex, (3) ventromedial prefrontal cortex, and (4) cingulate cortex. The dorsolateral prefrontal cortex is involved in what are known as 'cold' decisions, while the orbitofrontal cortex is important for 'hot' decision making. Anatomic orientation within the skull is provided.

The hot decision-making computer task involves betting on whether you think a golden token is hidden under a red or a blue box (there are ten boxes in total, of which a variable proportion are red or blue; see Figure 11). In each round of the game, the proportion of red and blue boxes changes, and each time, the computer randomly hides the token under one of these ten boxes. The participant can choose to bet 5 per cent, 25 per cent, 50 per cent, 75 per cent, or 95 per cent of his total points (representing money), and if he chooses the colour of the box hiding the token correctly, he wins that number of points. If he does not choose correctly, however, he loses those points. Most people do not like to risk losing money (even play money!), and so the game takes on an emotional component: happiness when

39

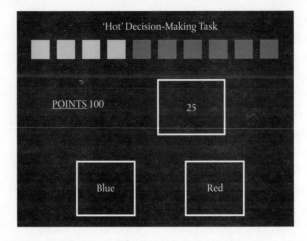

FIGURE 11 CANTAB Cambridge Gambling Task (www.camcog.com). The golden token is randomly hidden under a blue or red box. If you choose correctly you will win 25 points. If you are incorrect, you will lose 25 points from the 100 points that were already accrued. Is the coin more likely to be under a red or a blue box?

winning points, and displeasure when losing points. In some circumstances, the amount of money a volunteer is given for participating in the study is related to how many points he or she wins. As we discussed above in the section on risk aversion, subjects are generally more averse to losing an amount than they are happy to be winning that same amount, or corresponding gain [33]. This task has proven to be a valuable tool for engaging hot decision-making faculties in a controlled and reproducible manner.

Tasks like these may seem a very abstract way of engaging with real-world decision-making capabilities, but the reality is that we can draw some very interesting conclusions from such studies. For instance, one interesting thing that we have learned using the computer tasks described above is that entrepreneurs are highly adept at risk taking, and at decision making in general. Starting a business or backing a high-stakes decision requires a certain tolerance for risk, coupled with an ability to assess the probabilities and business realities involved. Research from our lab revealed that entrepreneurs and managers both make similar-quality cold decisions. In other words, they have similar baseline analytical skills. However, in the hot task, entrepreneurs showed an inclination to bet big—which, to be honest, is unusual for someone older than 30 years—whereas managers were much more conservative [34]. At the end of the study, the entrepreneurs had amassed a small fortune from bets, whereas the managers had not. Our study emphasized the importance of matching the correct decision-making skill set to a particular line of work. 'Functional impulsivity' is beneficial for seizing opportunities in a rapidly changing environment, or when opportunities are time limited. Successful entrepreneurs struck an appropriate balance between hot and cold decision making, as well as cognitive flexibility in problem solving, and were able to display superior performance on our computerized task. This same cognitive ability likely contributes to the success of these entrepreneurs in many business arenas. Now that we have a better understanding of the types of decisions that are needed, business training and education may be able to target these skills. *Forbes* magazine noted one potentially momentous consequence of this finding: "that training better hot decision-making is within the realm of possibility" [35].

We have touched on a few of the methods used by neuroscientists to open a window into the mind and investigate brain activity during certain tasks. There are still other methods used by neuroscientists—transcranial magnetic stimulation, tractography, single photon emission computed tomography—but they are used less frequently by neuroscientists than the methods discussed in this chapter. The sorts of odd neurological phenomena that usually get reported in the press—Maternal Instinct Is Wired Into the Brain [36], the brain's 'Buy Button'[37], the ability to see a person's intentions [38]—are just the tip of the iceberg of recent neuroscientific discoveries that have been made using these techniques.[31]

* * *

Now that we have reviewed some basics about how decisions are made and the methods that researchers and scientists use to assess brain function during decision-making tasks, we can turn to a crucial component of the decision-making process: the role of extreme emotions and medical pathologies. Simply put, a variety of emotional factors can affect decision making and degrade the quality of decisions that people make. These emotional factors range from normal moods to more extreme psychological conditions like mania and depression, and even further to neurological conditions that arise from trauma. Emotions are a critical component in decision making by both healthy and ill individuals, but it is in the extreme cases where their significance is most clearly defined, and the justification for interventional techniques is strongest.

3

EXTREME EMOTIONS AND RISKY BEHAVIOUR

I spent a lot of money on booze, birds and fast cars. The rest I just squandered.
George Best, football player

No passion so effectually robs the mind of all its powers of acting and reasoning as fear.   Edmund Burke, philosopher

Unhappy people do reckless things.   Cuddy, character in *House*, TV drama

It probably comes as no surprise that emotions have a direct and dramatic effect on decision making in particular, and behaviour more generally. This is common sense. When we are angry, or sad, or frustrated, we will tend to act in a certain way—indeed, the ways in which other people *act* are often the chief evidence we have about what they are *feeling*, and these actions can be far more revealing than a person's own explanations for a behaviour. So, the overall link between emotions and decisions is intuitively clear. But the mechanisms that link these two aspects are complex and are only now beginning to be understood.

Imagine that someone has irresponsibly swerved in front of your car and slammed on his brakes, and that in order to avoid a collision you also need to slam on your brakes and swerve. This stimulus results in neurochemical changes and the release of neurotransmitters—chemicals within your nervous system such as dopamine, serotonin, noradrenaline, and acetylcholine. These neuro-transmitters then propagate signals through your spinal cord to prompt a physiological reaction; in this case, to signal your adrenal glands to release adrenaline—or epinephrine, as it is called in the United States—into your bloodstream. The adrenaline travels to different parts of the body and results in what is known colloquially as a 'fight or flight' response. During a fight or flight response, your heart rate increases, pupils dilate, and your facial expressions and breathing patterns change; your sphincters tighten, mouth and eyes become dry, and blood vessels redirect blood to your muscles. Your body is preparing to fight or flee as the adrenaline coursing through it primes your muscles. In this way, the emotional state has prepared you to respond. Of course, the simple reality of having adrenaline in your system does not prompt a single type of response. Each person is affected differently, and the response is highly dependent on the situation.

Perhaps, if you are feeling enraged, you might roll down the window and yell at the person who caused such an unacceptable annoyance—that is, you might *fight*. On the other hand, perhaps you are a new driver, and so terrified that there was such a near miss that instead of experiencing anger that the irresponsible driver in front nearly caused an accident, you want to pull to the side of the road and recover—to *flee*. Another reaction might simply be relief. A given experience can produce different emotions, and influence our behaviour in different ways. Such an intense bodily reaction may also help you to recall these events more readily in the future. In other words, the emotion affects the formation and retention of a memory.

Let us pause for a minute: what of this word *emotion*? Before we get much further ahead of ourselves, we need to look more closely at what we mean by emotion. An initial working definition for emotion might be 'a reaction to an external stimulus that results in changes in our bodies to motivate behaviour'. But then again, emotions can be reactions to something internal as well. So we should revise our definition to something like this: emotions are reactions to events that trigger changes in our body's physiology and motivate our behaviour. For an emotion to occur it seems that chemicals are released, and these chemicals interact between neurons to produce an emotion.

It seems reasonable, then, to redefine emotions in terms of a neuronal response to a stimulus that results in the release of certain chemicals that change one's body and behaviour. We know that our bodies instinctively react to certain stimuli (for instance, shock or surprise) by making changes to neurochemistry that result in our being more suited for particular actions in response to that stimulus. The *emotions* we feel are a way of understanding these physiological reactions; they are labels we give to a reaction, not the reaction itself. The point at which and the manner in which one's body's reaction is labelled as a certain emotion—anger, fear, surprise—is largely unknown, as is how a certain emotion comes to be labelled as happiness, anger, and so on. Some theorize that emotions are learned reactions, and others claim that we are born with an innate set of core emotions—happiness, sadness, disgust, surprise, anger, and fear— and only some are learned.

The anatomy of an emotion is another elusive issue. As we mentioned above, the brain is divided into halves—a left hemisphere and a right hemisphere. Each hemisphere has a frontal, parietal, temporal, and occipital lobe, with some people also claiming that the insula represents a fifth lobe (see Figure 12). These lobes seem to be functionally distinct regions. The occipital lobe, for example, has an important role in visual processing, while the frontal lobe has an important role in decision making and planning (the so-called 'executive functions'), as well as other things such as initiating movement. The lobes communicate with each other via neuronal pathways, and scientists have identified pathways responsible for a variety of complex phenomena—including emotions. The limbic system, for example, connects the smelling centres, memory areas, fear and anger regions, reward and pleasure centres, decision-making and attention territories of the brain, and is thought to be responsible in large part for the regulation of emotions and emotionally charged memories.[1]

The road rage—if you succumbed to rolling down your window and yelling at the driver in front of you—is an example of how our emotions can play a part in our decision making. Surely, you would not have decided to roll the window down and yell if you were not upset. As we previously discussed, this sort of decision making is referred to as hot decision making.[2]

We are all familiar with situations when we have had to take a deep breath and count to ten to stop our emotions from getting the better of us, especially when contemplating important decisions for which we know that a cool and level head is best. Aren't these the times when we might take out a piece of paper and make a pro and con list in order to most objectively weigh two or more alternatives? Emotions sometimes interfere in our decisions, and some might argue that as far as most day-to-day decisions are concerned, the less emotion is involved, the more positive the outcome.

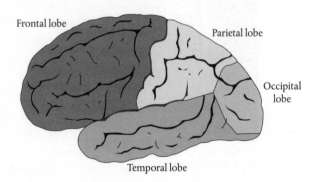

FIGURE 12 Basic diagram of the brain showing the four main lobes: frontal, parietal, occipital, and temporal.

Chess is a good example of a situation demanding high levels of logic, and minimal, preferably absent, amounts of emotion during a match. Garry Kasparov was world junior chess champion at the age of 16, and in 1985 at the age of 22, became the youngest world chess champion. His chess fame earned him an invitation to compete against an IBM computer named Deep Blue (see Figure 13) in 1996—a match that Kasparov won. However, computer technology was advancing at a prodigious rate, and it was not long before a computer could work through all logical outcomes of a game quite quickly. Kasparov was approached again by IBM in 1997 to compete against Deep Blue once more, and lost. When Kasparov aimed to explain his defeat, he cited the untoward influences of emotions—especially fear—and the pressure of the match; he—unlike Deep Blue—was emotionally vulnerable.[3]

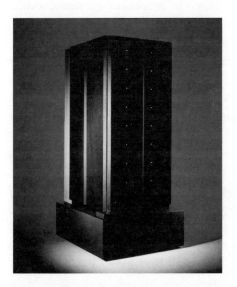

FIGURE 13 In 1996, Garry Kasparov beat IBM's Deep Blue computer at chess. In 1997, though, he lost a rematch.

Courtesy of International Business Machines Corporation, © International Business Machines Corporation.

Lest we give the cold and rational being too much credit, let us consider the manner in which emotional decision making can sometimes be a good thing. While it is certainly true that our emotions can occasionally make us behave in risky or bizarre ways, this is not to say that emotions should—or can—be avoided completely. Most basically, human society and interpersonal interactions are dependent on emotions. They enable our attraction to our partners, even after a few prior relationship debacles might have us thinking that such attraction is illogical. They also enable our ability to love and, in most cases, do almost anything for the benefit of our children. Emotions help us to be unpredictable, in a world where predictability may not be ideal. They often correspond to quite sophisticated and accurate judgements: a 'gut feeling' that something is right or wrong will often turn out to be correct, even if the reasoning process that led to this feeling cannot be articulated or reproduced.[4] Emotions are present at times and in ways that we might not think of as being emotional, and often keep us on track in our daily activities. A feeling of guilt, for instance, can be a huge motivator.

When we rouse from sleep, some of the most vestigial parts of the brain—the brainstem and thalamus—transmit their call for consciousness and arousal to 'higher' parts of the brain, the neocortex. Our dreamy trance fades, the world comes into view, and our thoughts (cognitions) and emotions rush into our heads. As we lie in our warm bed, perhaps we realize that it is raining outside and cold in the room; better to stay in bed. However, maybe we are looking forward to work, or perhaps we decide to get up because of a sense of duty and responsibility, and to alleviate the inevitable sense of guilt that would arise if we decided to stay in bed longer and arrive late for work. Whenever we are making decisions, emotions are almost certainly in the background. The pathways between supposedly non-emotional decision making and those areas specialized for emotional processing interact in ways that allow our rational selves to be influenced by our emotions, and vice versa. This critical interaction is necessary for normal life.

As nice as it would be to take credit for the idea that emotions and rationality might be separable parts of our being, we cannot. Over 2,000 years ago, Plato proposed that there were distinct components to decision making in humans. He argued that when faced with decisions we feel the pull of different forces in different directions, causing us ultimately to lean towards one way or the other. As the centrepiece of his *Phaedrus*, Plato provides an analogy of the soul as a charioteer with two winged horses. One horse was upright and cleanly made, while the other was powerful and unruly. We can adapt Plato's moral analogy slightly and think of the upright horse as representing rational decision making, while the powerful unruly horse represents emotional decision making. The charioteer who attempts to control these two animals is ultimately dependent upon and driven by them—much like our own consciousness—and only in unison can the composite function effectively. The notion that emotions can interfere with decision making is not just ancient philosophical stuff, nor is it an unusual circumstance.

We are a complicated species, and our emotional states are far from static, as we can quickly see when we try to describe even the simplest emotions in detail. Consider happiness. Generally, happiness and sadness are considered polar opposites, set in accepted opposition to each other, but in fact they form a continuum, called the affective (mood) spectrum (see Figure 14). When we think of our emotional state in these terms, it is not that we are turning one emotion off (e.g. sad) and another on (e.g. happy). Rather, our emotional state can at any time be described as somewhere along the continuum between happy and sad. The other core emotions (fear, surprise, anger, and disgust) affect us in similar ways, although it is more

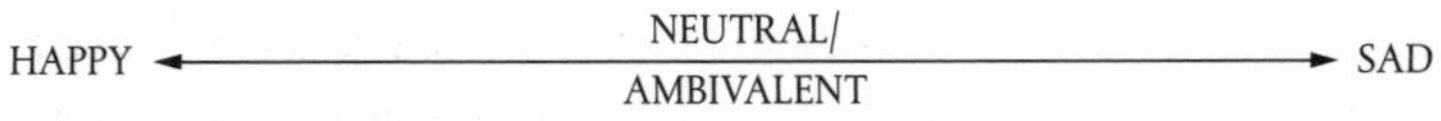

HAPPY ◄─────────── NEUTRAL/ ───────────► SAD
                   AMBIVALENT

FIGURE 14 The affective mood spectrum places happy and sad at opposite ends of a continuum.

49

difficult to conceptualize them as a continuum.[5] The reader certainly knows from personal experience that there are varying degrees of these emotions ranging from neutral through to whatever maximum extreme might be possible (e.g. absolute terror). Each emotion exists on a continuum, and the varying states along these continua ultimately contribute to the overall mood. In terms of decisions, our emotions become more or less influential depending on where along these continua we lie at any given time.

On a daily basis most people fluctuate within a central 'normal' region of the continuum (see Figure 15). Perhaps, if you have recently been promoted or have fallen in love, your mood is towards the happy end. In fact, reading the previous sentence may have reminded you about a pleasant experience and you had a transient shift along the continuum still further towards happy. Alternatively, if you have recently suffered a loss, your mood might be headed off towards the sad end of the spectrum. It is important to realize that we all experience these fluctuations in mood and they are not the same thing as existing continuously on the polar extremes. Individuals usually exist on the slightly more positive side of the continuum, which may confer a certain degree of resilience if something stressful or unpleasant were to happen [39]. In fact, it might be that we are resilient against extremes of mood largely *because* they exert an inordinate influence over decision making, leading to behaviours that we realize may have catastrophic consequences. Once one spends some time at an emotional extreme, it becomes more difficult to break out of this state and return to a 'normal' emotional state.

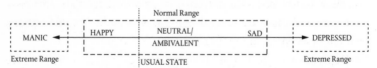

FIGURE 15 The affective mood spectrum extends to extreme ranges, usually considered maladaptive. Most people exist around a central 'normal' region of the continuum just slightly towards the happy end, thus conferring resilience.

While many of us feel down from time to time, this does not stop us from getting up in the morning, or from going to work and being reasonably productive; these occasional mood slumps are not the same as clinical depression. Depression is one extreme end of the spectrum, and although it is quite common, it is not a normal reaction to any situation. We cannot 'snap' someone out of clinical depression. At this extreme, the emotion has a pervasive and inescapable influence on the person's decisions and actions.

The intensity of this emotional state, and its dissimilarity from normal swings of mood, highlights one difficulty in accurately diagnosing and categorizing it, and in helping patients to recognize it. How might we assess the emotional state of a given individual, i.e. the position that an individual occupies on the various emotional continua? The most straightforward method is simply to ask the person to, for example, mark a cross on a line somewhere between 'not at all' and 'as much as possible' to describe each component of their emotional state at that moment in time. However, the self-reported survey method has the real drawback that a person can only rate what he or she is feeling based on past experience. Unless someone has experienced it himself, most people cannot truly conceive of a mood so low that they neither want to eat nor interact with people, a sadness so encompassing that they cannot be motivated to take care of children and would rather die. Therefore, psychiatrists have had to devise measures and specific criteria to judge whether someone's emotional state is actually beyond 'normal', even if that someone is the saddest he has ever been, and can ever imagine being. These criteria allow us to discuss the extremes of emotion in a relatively objective way, and there are several well-known conditions that affect a patient's placement along the emotional spectrum.

Depression is the first psychiatric and medical condition that we will consider—and since an estimated 9.1 per cent (nearly 1 in 10) of US adults suffer from some form of depression,[6] it is sadly familiar to many. The symptoms are quite diverse, but to be diagnosed with clinical (unipolar) depression, a person must have a depressed or irritable mood—among other things—that persists for weeks at a time without experiencing any highs.[7] The author William Styron called depression "a sensation close to, but indescribably different from, actual pain" that healthy people usually cannot understand, "due not to a failure of sympathy but to the basic inability of healthy people to imagine a form of torment so alien to everyday experience" [40]. However, it is not just that the person feels down; he may also report a lack of energy, difficulty getting started in the morning, a loss of interest in friends as well as activities that he previously enjoyed, guilt, sleep and appetite disturbances, or thoughts of wanting to die.[8] The symptoms of depression are relatively well understood,[9] even though the causes are not. No particular cause seems to apply to every patient.

Consider that some people have tragic childhoods and early life experiences: abuse—emotional, physical, psychological—by family, friends, and strangers, or they observe catastrophic events such as parents or a partner dying. Not everyone with these experiences goes on to develop depression, but some do. Also consider that some people grow up in ostensibly loving households and have what appear to be valuable childhood experiences, but as adults they suffer from chronic long-term depression without any apparent cause. The aetiology of depression is complicated and difficult to understand, but surely involves an interaction between genes and environment, as well as an interaction between traits of resilience and genetic predisposition to depression.

Depression is not confined to particular social classes, and certainly has its famous sufferers. Sir Winston Churchill (see Figure 16a) famously spoke of his depression as his "black dog", providing a powerful metaphor for the experience:

> I think this man might be useful to me – if my black dog returns. He seems quite away from me now – it is such a relief. All the colours come back into the picture.[10]

Churchill perhaps got the phrase from reading Sir Walter Scott's journals:

Something of the black dog still hanging about me; but I will shake him off. I generally affect good spirits in company of my family, whether I am enjoying them or not [41].[11]

Other great men—and women—have suffered from periods of depression; it is thought that Goethe—author of *Faust* and a man who would influence later scientific, musical, literary, and poetic thought—was a sufferer, as was Abraham Lincoln (see Figure 16b):

I am now the most miserable man living. If what I feel were equally distributed to the whole human family, there would not be one cheerful face on the earth. Whether I shall ever be

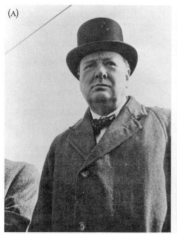
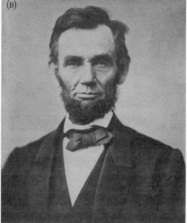

FIGURE 16 A) Sir Winston Churchill and B) President Abraham Lincoln both suffered from depression. Many famous and successful people have lived with depression.

(A) Winston Churchill, c. 1942. Library of Congress, LC-USW33-019093-C ; (B) Abraham Lincoln, 1863, Library of Congress, LC-DIG-ppmsca-19301

better I can not tell; I awfully forebode I shall not. To remain as
I am is impossible; I must die or be better, it appears to me.[12]

Leo Tolstoy, Hans Christian Anderson, Mary Shelley, the comedian
Rodney Dangerfield—the list goes on. Certainly, Churchill was in
distinguished company.

The presence of so many popular creative individuals listed
above—and also below when we discuss bipolar disorder—is
striking. It has been said that:

> Mental illness does not necessarily cause creativity, nor does
> creativity necessarily contribute to mental illness, but a certain
> ruminating personality type may contribute to both mental
> health issues and art [42].

Many studies have looked at the association between creativity and
mood disorders over the years, and there does seem to be a relationship. A recent study by a group of researchers from Syracuse, New
York investigated the link between depressive symptoms and a
propensity towards a self-reflective nature. Those who were more
ruminative were felt to have objectively increased creative fluency
[43]. One of the researchers for this project notes that:

> If you think about stuff in your life and you start thinking about
> it again, and again, and again, and you kind of spiral away in this
> continuous rumination about what's happening to you and to
> the world—people who do that are at risk for depression [42].

This propensity towards continuous rumination, particularly if rumi-
nating about something negative, is an important focus of cognitive
behavioural therapy, which is based largely on the work of Aaron Beck.

Aaron Beck's cognitive model of depression proposed that an individual's mood distorted the way in which people viewed the world,
which in turn affected self-esteem, decision making, and actions,
which then served to reinforce and conflate the negative mood—a

sort of emotional Catch-22.[13] Beck claimed that the abnormal cognitions (thoughts) were just as integral to depression as the low mood itself. To his mind, it was not just extreme emotions that mattered; what mattered most was how emotion and thoughts interacted.

According to his theory, our framework (schema) for interpreting the world is with us from a very early age, and affects our interpretation of information that we collect about the world and our role in it. If one's schema is negatively biased, that individual is more inclined to perceive things in a negative light. Rogue negative schemata can become activated at any point in life, and once activated they can then lead to systematic errors. For instance, people with depression tend to repeatedly overlook positive experiences and compliments that people give them, but spend a great amount of time cogitating on even minor setbacks or criticisms; they fixate on the negative, directing this negativity towards themselves, the world, and the future. Because the source of the problem is thought to be a person's framework of interpretation, cognitive behavioural therapy is directed at changing the depressed individual's cognitions.[14] In this way, cognitive behavioural therapy allows the frontal cortices to exert a type of top-down processing over areas that are important for emotional regulation and interpretation [44].

Mania is at the other end of the affective spectrum. Mania is very different from the happiness that most of us experience in response to pleasant and exciting life events, or even the 'high' that athletes get from exercise. When people suffer from manic episodes they have an abnormally elated mood that persists for at least one week. This elated mood, which in and of itself might be pleasurable or addictive, is damaging in other ways. Just as with extreme negative mood, intense positive moods can influence our decisions and actions for the worse, to the detriment of everyday life. Typically, people with mania talk very quickly and have ideas that fly so rapidly through their minds that what they say may make only fragmented sense to a listener. The manic patient finds it difficult to concentrate and his attention is easily drawn to things that shouldn't matter or that are irrelevant. They might sleep for as little as two or three hours per night, compared with the typical seven or eight. Mania can also lead to risky behaviour that may seem exciting or fun, but that leads to damaging consequences. For instance, the manic patient may gamble away his life savings, spend wildly on his credit cards during a shopping spree, make bizarre and risky business decisions, or drive at breakneck speed on busy roads. This behaviour is often worsened by the tendency for manic individuals to think that they are special or unique in some way, have special powers, or feel that they can do things that no one else can do. Stories of manic cases show up time and time again in psychiatric literature.

For instance, there was a quiet man who woke up one morning believing that he had discovered a way to keep fish alive forever. He withdrew the family savings, spent it all on aquatic equipment, and planned to travel to the USA to find willing customers for his amazing invention [45]. Another case report presented a 38-year-old woman who on the day prior to her second admission to the hospital for manic symptoms purchased fifty-seven hats [46]. These stories seem incredible, but the excess positive emotions expressed by the person can be extremely convincing, and amazing tales of heroic flight and fancy may also regale observers. It is often only after speaking with a relative who knows the manic individual well that it becomes clear that something is wrong.

Other individuals move between manic states and intense depression. This existence, cycling—perhaps quickly, perhaps slowly—between the two poles of the affective spectrum, is what is known as bipolar disorder.[15]

Just as there is a lengthy list of famous individuals suffering from unipolar depression, there is also a plethora of distinguished sufferers of bipolar disorder. Lord Byron was described by Lady Caroline Lamb as "mad, bad, and dangerous to know".[16] His fame comes from his life in addition to his poetry, as he was reported to live extravagantly, had numerous love affairs and extramarital exploits, and found himself often in debt—all examples of the reckless and risky behaviour seen in manic patients. There are many others: Charles Dickens, Ralph Waldo Emerson, William Faulkner, F. Scott Fitzgerald, and Stephen Fry, for example. The researcher Kay Redfield Jamison has compiled a list of possible bipolar sufferers in her various books, and suffers from bipolar disorder herself.[17]

As we mentioned above, there are many different emotions along different spectra. Fear is an example of an emotion very different from sadness or happiness. Most individuals can name something of which they are afraid. For instance, spiders often induce fear; many people dislike spiders and the way they move, the way they may appear in shrubs and hidden in corners of houses. However, when most people see a spider—even though they may feel upset or even uncomfortable—they do not suffer physical symptoms of extreme anxiety, such as sweating, dizziness, heart palpitations, muscle tension, trembling, a dry mouth, nausea, and an impending sense of doom. This physical manifestation of fear is known as a *panic attack*, and can accompany severe *phobias*, which are intense yet irrational fears of certain things, situations, activities, or people. There are numerous phobias, and anyone can have a phobia of almost anything (see Table 1 for a selection of some common and not-so-common phobias).

Individuals with a phobia suffer overpowering fear and anxiety; they can sometimes barely think of the object of their fears without instigating a panic attack. In some circumstances, people come to fear the panic attack almost as much as the object of their initial fears, so that the anxiety about the panic attack itself sparks a panic attack, which then sparks more anxiety, and the vicious cycle continues unabated.[18]

It is easy to see how such an extreme emotion can have a huge impact on decision making. Imagine for an instant that you are afraid of public speaking—one form of a social phobia. However, your boss asks you to do a presentation about your company's assets.

TABLE I A selection of common and not-so-common phobias

Phobia	Fear of:
Ablutophobia	Bathing, washing, and cleaning
Acrophobia	Heights
Aerophobia	Flying
Agoraphobia	Any place or situation where escape might be difficult or help unavailable in the event of developing sudden panic-like symptoms, especially open spaces
Amaxophobia	Driving or riding in vehicles
Androphobia	Coming into contact, engaging in activities, or becoming intimate with men
Arachibutyrophobia	Peanut butter sticking to the roof of one's mouth
Apiphobia	Bees
Arachnophobia	Spiders
Automatonophobia	Anything that falsely represents a sentient being, including ventriloquist dummies, animatronic creatures, or wax statues
Bacteriophobia	Contamination and germs
Barophobia	Gravity
Brontophobia	Thunderstorms
Chrematophobia	Money
Claustrophobia	Being trapped in small confined spaces
Consecotaleophobia	Chopsticks
Dextrophobia/Levophobia	The right/left side of the body
Eisoptrophobia	Mirrors, or seeing one's reflection
Enetophobia	Being around sharp objects, being stuck by a needle or pin
Epistaxiophobia	Nosebleeds

Phobia	Fear of:
Ergophobia	Work environment (assigned tasks, speaking before groups at work, or socializing with co-workers)
Geniophobia	Chins
Gephyrophobia	Bridges
Glossophobia	Having to express oneself in front of a group of people; speaking
Gymnophobia	Nudity
Gynophobia	Women
Hematophobia	Losing, giving, receiving or just seeing blood
Hippopotomonstrosesquipedaliophobia	Long words
Homophobia	Homosexuality
Hydrophobia	Water
Iatrophobia	Any person who performs surgery, administers shots, gives medical diagnostics, or any others in the medical field
Ideophobia	New or different ideas, or fear of thought
Microphobia	Germs
Necrophobia	Death or dead things
Obesophobia	Gaining weight; often seen in anorexia and bulimia
Odontophobia	Teeth
Paralipophobia	Neglect or omission of some duty
Paraskavedekatriaphobia	The number 13 (and Friday the 13th in particular)
Pediophobia	A child or doll
Peladophobia	Becoming bald or of being around bald people

(*continued*)

TABLE I (*continued*)

Phobia	Fear of:
Pentheraphobia	The mother-in-law
Phobophobia	Developing a phobia, or the fear of fear
Phonemophobia	Thinking, or one's own thoughts
Pteronophobia	Being tickled by others or by feathers
Somniphobia	Sleep and that once asleep the sufferer may not wake up again
Urophobia	The act of urinating in a public rest room, of hearing others urinating, or of urine itself; often linked with social phobias

Even if you suspect there is nothing to worry about, even if you think that you have valuable information on the topic, even if you would like to be able to do such a presentation, the fear of being in the limelight (and being evaluated and possibly negatively judged) brings with it such a tremendous amount of anxiety that your heart begins to palpitate, your palms become clammy, and you become light-headed, and you really feel that if you have to fulfil your public role, you might just die. Not only do you retreat from the situation, you actively avoid your boss so he cannot ask you again. Then perhaps you begin to avoid work altogether. If your boss does find you to ask you again, perhaps you call in sick on the day of the would-be presentation. This is different from just being shy; in the case of a phobia, one's behaviour is driven and controlled by fear.

Nearly 10 per cent of the individuals reading the preceding description will find the scenario familiar, as social phobia is the most common phobia.[19] Not only is this phobia different from mere shyness, it can be present in people who function quite well in certain public roles. For instance, when Kim Basinger stood up to accept her Best Supporting Actress award for her performance in *LA Confidential*, she was apparently so terrified that she forgot the words to her acceptance speech, even though she had been practising for days.

Generally, individuals with social phobia undervalue their worth and underestimate their social skills and abilities; they tend to see negative reactions in other people, which distract them from focusing and seeing positive feedback. These negative cognitions are reminiscent of Beck's cognitive model of depression. As such, therapy for phobias is aimed at restructuring an individual's experiences with the object of their fear; an individual is meant to unlearn the conditioned response that resulted in fear in the first place. Desensitization therapy, as it is called, can be very successful, and as people move through the therapy they learn to conquer anxiety-provoking situations with relaxation techniques and by adopting new cognitions.[20]

It is not only extreme emotions that may cause problems in cognitive function generally and decision making in particular. A lack of emotion or inability to recognize the emotions of others may also affect one's functioning. These are termed problems of social cognition. In fact, Asperger's syndrome—which is a developmental disorder identifiable in childhood—is diagnosed partly because of social awkwardness, or an inability to emotionally interact with other individuals. In other words, these children lack the ability to read and communicate emotional cues, despite average or above-average intellect. The child is aware of missing something in social interaction, but is unable to understand how another person might be feeling, why someone behaves in a particular way, or another's intentions. Social reciprocity—the idea that if you help me out, then I'll help you out—is also often lost. It should be noted that these children are still able to feel and express emotions, such as frustration or anger, but are unable to form normal emotional connections with other individuals, even their family, friends, and caregivers.

The way in which people attribute mental states to the self and others is usually known as the theory of mind, and it may have some basis in the recently discovered 'mirror neurons'—these are neurons that become excited when we watch people behave in certain ways, promoting imitation and perhaps empathy. This 'mirroring' action means that observing a particular emotional state or behaviour essentially triggers that same state or behaviour in ourselves.[21] Professor Vilayanur Ramachandran from the University of California at San Diego has suggested that these neurons may be involved in complex behaviours such as imitation. Others suggest that mirror neurons may be involved in language acquisition and theory of mind skills. Whatever the origin, one aspect of the theory of mind that is often under-recognized is that our understanding of emotion allows us to understand and even predict behaviour in other people: for instance, when we think to ourselves, 'Oh, he's upset, so he'll probably _____', or, 'She's embarrassed, so now she will _____'. This type of empathetic understanding is amazingly subtle, and in some sense, this makes us all 'mind readers', but it is so commonplace that we don't realize how remarkable it actually is. However, it depends on a very intuitive and thorough understanding of the relationship between emotions and decisions. The continual presence of this understanding in our own consciousness is perhaps one of the reasons why the behaviour associated with extreme emotions is so difficult to predict—we simply don't expect it because the underlying pathological emotions are unknown to us.

Some scientists believe that the development of theory of mind skills begins at a very young age, even before an infant walks. As development continues, a child will come to use body language and verbal language in a way that brings about a desired outcome. However, children with autism and autistic spectrum disorders (such as Asperger's syndrome) tend to have difficulties with theory of mind skills. Imagine how difficult it might be to interact with someone if you could not attribute desires and emotions to them.[22] Our perception of people's thoughts and feelings guides our behaviour on a daily basis, and it is easy to take this ability for granted. But the next time you are able to perceive that someone is not *really* that interested in your lecture or conversation, consider how your behaviour might change if you could only understand the transcript and not the subtext...if you could not read people and situations.

Up until this point, we have spent time discussing conditions that generally present themselves before midlife. Now let us look at two types of dementia, which generally develop in later life: Alzheimer's disease and frontotemporal dementia, which are alike in that they both produce cognitive difficulties. However, they also result in aberrant emotional responses, and the decision-making difficulties that people suffering from these disorders experience are thought to be a result of a combination of emotional difficulty and cognitive difficulty.

Alzheimer's disease continues to become more prevalent as the world's population ages, and the United States has over five million sufferers of the disease. The probability of being diagnosed with Alzheimer's disease is approximately 2–5 per cent at age 65, and doubles every five years thereafter [47]; in fact, by the year 2040 the global prevalence is expected to reach 81 million elderly individuals [48].[23] This disease is characterized at first by problems in episodic memory function—remembering where one parked one's car in a multilevel car park several hours before, or remembering where one left one's house keys the previous evening—as the hippocampal formation within the temporal lobes is affected (see Figure 17).[24] In these early stages, patients retain their social grace and are fairly adept at covering up their difficulties. In later stages, the disease is characterized by personality changes and emotionally variable states as its neuropathological process begins to affect other brain areas including the frontal lobes. Patients are often confused and become irritable, agitated, anxious, or fearful, which can be attributed to the fact that they often suspect that something may be happening—but may not know or understand the specifics—and they are also aware that they can no longer compensate for their deficits. Alternatively, they can become apathetic and placid. Patients may withdraw from social interaction and family.

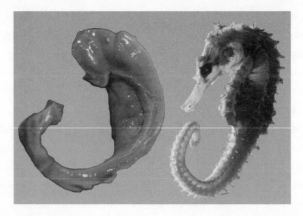

FIGURE 17 The hippocampus is intimately involved in memory formation, and 'hippocampus' is the Latin name for seahorse. Here we have a preparation of the hippocampus alongside a seahorse, as done by László Seress.

Courtesy of Professor László Seress

Long-term memory—remembering one's grandchildren and children, or remembering that one's spouse has passed away—is traditionally thought to be affected nearer the end of a disease process that can last from five to fifteen years prior to death.

On the other hand, frontotemporal dementia (FTD) affects personality and emotional health first, and subsequently affects memory as the disease progresses. This reflects the anatomy of the disease, which begins in the frontal lobes of the brain, and eventually involves the temporal lobe. However, since the episodic memory systems largely involve the hippocampus (in the temporal lobes), memory function remains relatively intact during the beginning of the disease. This disease is more common than most people think, and one of every seven patients with dementia has FTD. Put another way, 15 of 100,000 people between the ages of 45 and 64 are thought to suffer from FTD [49].[25] These are patients who are affected at an earlier age than patients with Alzheimer's disease, at a time when they are in the prime of their working lives and may still have young families. They are usually identified because of an early change in personal or social conduct. FTD patients can be apathetic and withdrawn—contrary to their prior behaviours—or show a disinhibition that can result in inappropriate or impulsive behaviour (swearing, outbursts, social tactlessness, shoplifting, shopping sprees, sexual indiscretions). They have repetitive behaviours, bizarre moods and emotions, and language disturbances.[26] In some ways, they behave similarly to manic patients.

As we will see shortly, both classes of demented patients discussed above usually have difficulties with 'executive functions', which are served by areas of the frontal lobes.

The brain basis of poor decision making

We have briefly outlined a selection of disorders in which extremes of emotion (or lack of emotional awareness) can result in abnormal decision making and other behaviours. Although the specific mechanisms are not yet understood, all of these changes in behaviour and decision making seem to be the result of different changes in brain chemistry and brain activity.[27]

Using a variety of techniques such as functional MRI, researchers are now beginning to elucidate the brain basis of these neuropsychiatric conditions. Understanding the brain functionality that accompanies particular types of abnormal decision making is not the whole story, but it is the first step towards helping the many people who suffer from conditions that affect their decision making.

The conditions we discussed above are prevalent but still relatively uncommon in absolute terms. Most people do not suddenly decide to go on ruinous spending sprees or go on holiday with a complete stranger. Nor do they gamble far beyond their financial limits, or hop on a motorcycle and drive at 140 mph on the M25 around London at four o'clock in the morning. They also do not usually jump off the tops of buildings because they think that they can fly or try to replicate the stunt jumps they've seen in action movies. But some people do. These individuals have lost the ability to fully evaluate

BAD MOVES

consequences or to connect those consequences to their own lives; they are incapable of applying, or decide to ignore, the basic piece of advice that accompanies most depictions of risky behaviour: *Don't try this at home*. For many of those suffering from mania, logical considerations based on accurate assessments are—at least transiently—impaired. 'I can do it!' is the order of the day...until they cannot.

Risky decisions can be successful or unsuccessful. Morality and philosophy aside, cognitively 'abnormal' decisions are dangerous or have the disproportionate potential to harm the individual. It is well known that some psychiatric and neurologic patients seem to make a disproportionate number of risky decisions—decisions that deviate from normal decision making. These patient cases might seem extreme, and they are, but by examining the most extreme cases we can get at the heart of an issue with relevance to us all: why do people make bad choices?

The reader may recall that mania and depression are defined by various characteristics and criteria. In mania, an individual has a feeling of enormous elation, doesn't require much sleep, makes lots of plans for the future, and is easily distracted. One of the most recognizable symptoms of mania, however, is that the individual participates in risk taking and impulsive behaviours, such as spending one's life savings on an unsound investment. Depressed individuals, on the other hand, often have trouble making up their minds or deciding a course of action; they are particularly *indecisive* or apathetic.

The kinds of patterns of decision making seen in mania and depression—risky decisions and indecision—are abnormal patterns of decision making. In fact, in many cases these decision-making patterns *define* the psychiatric condition. In other words, making poor quality or maladaptive decisions that impair functioning is one thing that differentiates the manic person from the merely energetic or elated individual. But this general observation begs the question: what sorts of patterns of decision making can we find in particular conditions, and more intriguingly, *why* are people with certain diagnoses predictably worse at making certain decisions?

Currently, our best method of investigating the function of different parts of the brain during decision making is to employ one or more of the methods we discussed in Chapter 2, all of which allow scientists to peer into the brain. These methods certainly have their limits, but they do allow us an unprecedented level of precision when talking about brain function, and have allowed us to learn quite a bit about decision making in psychiatric and neurological populations.

The first particular point we have learned is that we should focus on a part of the brain known as the prefrontal cortex, which is best thought of as the most forward part of the brain. This prefrontal brain region is subdivided into main divisions and other additional areas. The main divisions are the orbitofrontal cortex (including parts of the ventromedial cortex) and dorsolateral prefrontal cortex; the other areas include the ventrolateral prefrontal cortex, anterior prefrontal cortex, and connections with the anterior cingulate. The prefrontal brain is referred to using precise and complicated terminology, and for a visual summary of the important terms, see Figure 18. The areas that are relevant to our discussion of decision making are just two: the orbitofrontal and dorsolateral cortices.

You may remember the terms orbitofrontal and dorsolateral from Chapter 2. The orbitofrontal cortex is (not surprisingly) the area of the brain towards the front and above the orbits of your eyes, while the dorsolateral cortex is the towards the top and to the side of each frontal lobe (see Figure 10). As we discussed in Chapter 2, the orbitofrontal and dorsolateral areas are involved in hot and cold decisions, respectively. Based on the most current research, we believe that the orbitofrontal cortex plays an important role in emotional, hot decision making, while the dorsolateral cortex is more involved in rational, non-emotional, cold decision making.

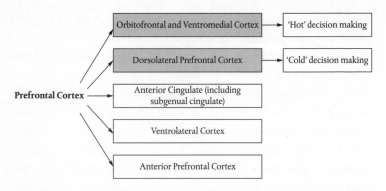

FIGURE 18 The prefrontal cortex is composed of main divisions (in grey) and three additional areas. The orbitofrontal cortex is known to be important for 'hot' decision making, whereas the dorsolateral prefrontal cortex is involved in 'cold' decision making.

The research into conditions that affect these areas is still in its infancy—and we will review it in due course—but we can already draw a few striking conclusions about the roles that these areas play in decision making, and what happens when normal function is interrupted. In patients who display difficulty with either hot or cold decisions, the functionality of these areas is abnormal. This seems to be true of both psychiatric and neurologic patients, though most research to date has focused on psychiatric patients, and in particular those patients with mania and depression.

On the one hand, this is a tremendously exciting and promising development in neuroscience. We have long understood that certain areas of the brain control particular functions—moving a limb or calculating how many 50-pence pieces are in three quid, for example. But something like decision making is infinitely more complex. Now we are beginning to be able to draw qualitative links between specific regions of the brain and a normative or non-normative ability for the patient to make beneficial decisions.

This tells us much ... but it also tells us next to nothing. Are neurological and psychiatric conditions the cause of such altered brain function, or are they a symptom of it? Is the reality (as we suspect) much more complicated than either cause or effect? These questions will undoubtedly drive the next generation of inquiry and discovery, and are a constant sobering reminder of how little we actually know about ourselves and the processes that make us. Inside each of our heads is the most complex structure in the known universe, and neuroscientific research has to grapple with that reality.

But in keeping one eye firmly on the promise and possibility of future research, we should not neglect what has been learned. And current research indicates a fascinating and surprising connection between well-recognized pathologies and well-defined difficulties in decision making.

Brain changes in mania and depression

In patients with depression and mania, the orbitofrontal (hot) and dorsolateral (cold) prefrontal cortices both show abnormal activity.

Think back to Chapter 2 when we discussed how PET scanning allows researchers to see which brain areas are 'turned on' and which are 'turned off'. Scientists can evaluate brain activity after providing the patient with a particular emotional stimulus. In these situations, the patient views an emotionally laden stimulus (such as a picture) while researchers look at their brain using PET or fMRI scans.

When emotionally charged stimuli are used, researchers see even more profound differences between individuals with psychiatric diagnoses and those without. For instance, when depressed patients look at positively charged (happy) or neutral pictures, their brain activity decreases in the orbitofrontal and cingulate areas—the parts of their brains involved in hot decision making. But when they view *sad* stimuli, these same parts of their brains become more active [50]. What is the significance of these findings? The increased brain activity indicates that, compared with healthy volunteers, the depressed patients are more aware of the sad stimuli. To a depressed patient, the sad stimulus is a stronger distraction that commands more of their attention than the happy stimulus does. And if their attention is grabbed, then they need to consciously suppress or inhibit that attention in order to make a decision or respond to a task, which takes time and effort.[28] This phenomenon could partly explain the difficulty that many depressed patients exhibit with making decisions, or their general tendency towards indecisiveness. To put it crudely, they are continually distracted by negative emotions that a non-depressed person would find easier to overlook.

Patients experiencing a manic episode, on the other hand, show increased brain activity in response to *happy* stimuli; their attention is *grabbed* by happy (as opposed to sad) words. The biases in attention of depressed patients to sad stimuli and manic patients to happy stimuli are known as mood congruent biases. They make intuitive sense given the extremely happy or sad moods the patients are exhibiting at the time. However, the crucial point with respect to decision making is that these biases affect a patient's ability to respond appropriately and/or in a timely fashion to the tasks at hand [51]. We know from Chapter 2 that the prefrontal brain is involved in decision making, and now we also know that depressed and manic patients both show abnormal brain activity in the same brain regions. Thus, it may not be surprising that these patients have difficulties with decision making.

Intriguingly, the orbitofrontal areas have connections with the limbic system, which is involved in emotional processing. Studies of depressed patients have shown that these patients feature increased blood flow in the almond-shaped area of the limbic system known as the amygdala [52]. The amygdala is thought to play an important role in emotional reactions (especially fear) and emotional memory. This means that the emotional circuit of the brain was activated or 'turned on' in depressed patients. Researchers also noted that depressive symptoms were positively correlated with blood flow—in other words, the amount of increased blood flow was related to how depressed a person reported feeling. Patients who reported feeling more depressed demonstrated more blood flow in that area.

Another study found that an area of the limbic system contained within the ventromedial prefrontal cortex—the subgenual (or anterior) cingulate[29]—is abnormally activated during episodes of mania and depression, and that treatment of the depression results in a normalization of the brain activation [53].[30] This study looked at resting brain activity, i.e. brain activity when the patient was not asked to perform a task, which means that the differences in blood flow or 'activation' existed in the absence of anything external to the patient; the differences were intrinsic to the brains of patients with these conditions.

The studies we have just discussed help explain the brain areas that depression and mania seem to affect, and they give some insight into why these patients have difficulty making decisions. These studies established important groundwork, but they say little about the *sorts* of difficulties that such patients have. More recent studies have begun to explore these questions.

How is decision making affected in mania and depression?

Think back to the Cambridge Gambling Task discussed in Chapter 2. This task is designed to test emotionally charged decision making, and we have found that it activates the orbitofrontal cortex, which is thought to be involved in hot decisions. Using this hot task, we have been able to confirm certain findings in patients who display characteristics of extreme emotions. For instance, depressed and manic patients take longer to respond on the Cambridge Gambling Task, i.e. they take longer to make decisions [54]—a finding congruent with the explanation that such patients are abnormally distracted. A similar pattern of decision difficulties is also seen in bipolar patients who are experiencing an episode of depression [55]—they take longer to make decisions. Average response time is a crude measurement, but it is also a well-established way of quantifying the complex idea that a patient is distracted by particular thoughts, and needs to suppress those thoughts in order to make a decision.

However, we can go beyond this initial metric to assess the quality—or lack thereof—of the decisions they do make. It is important to reiterate that terms like 'bad' or 'high quality' or 'harmful' are not meant to carry any moral force. We are not making a moral claim here. What we mean by bad decisions is that these are decisions that are less likely to achieve the aims that are explained to the patients in the experiment. For instance, patients with mania make risky bets and wager more liberally (i.e. they use suboptimal betting strategies), both of which tend to decrease their overall winnings over the course of the experiment [54]. Manic patients also tend to choose the less probable of two options (i.e. they frequently bet on the 'underdog'). By contrast, even though depressed individuals may take risks, they still choose the more favourable of two options, whereas manic patients do not [54].

It also seems that as patients have more severe episodes of mania, the quality of their decision making decreases. In a similar way, depressed individuals who have attempted suicide perform worse on a gambling task than non-depressed individuals [56]. They also perform worse compared with other depressed individuals who have not attempted suicide. In fact, this poor decision making may be one of the things that make suicide attempts more prevalent among the depressed patient population. The chain of experiences that informs a decision to take one's own life is tragic. A compliment is quickly forgotten but an innocent question is regarded as a criticism and obsessed over for days. That individual loses interest in recreational activities, in any sort of fulfilling work, in loved ones and pets, in music and cinema, in travel and food. The experiences of life are drained of all savour and become worthless. To someone in that condition, the decision to take his or her life is, in a narrow sense, tragically understandable—it might be the only decision they can think to make when confronted with a day-to-day experience that seems unbearable and unlikely ever to improve.

Manic patients also make poorer-quality decisions when their symptoms are more severe [54]. It is important to remember that risky behaviour encompasses a large number and variety of categories, not just decisions that result in physical harm.[31] These experiments do investigate a very limited and controlled set of decisions, but nevertheless the real-life implications of these findings are huge. Imagine what sort of benefit could be seen in someone whose psychiatric condition is appropriately managed and optimally treated. Furthermore, a crucial practical step in managing these conditions can simply be for physicians and psychologists to encourage patients to recognize their condition, and not to make life-changing decisions during episodes when their symptoms are strongest. Patients who ignore this advice often come to regret their decisions—or, worse, die as a result of them.

These patterns of poor decision making in depressed and manic patients are seen as early as the teenage years. During their first episode of depression, adolescents, like adults, bet impulsively, especially during more difficult decisions. They are also biased to recognize and categorize things as being sad more frequently than happy; they have a bias towards negative or sad stimuli and are 'primed towards negativity' [57].

Up until now, we have discussed emotional decision making, and reviewed some of the evidence indicating how it is affected in mania and depression. Cold decision making is a different class entirely, although manic and depressed patients also often display deficits in cold decision making.

The Stockings of Cambridge task discussed in Chapter 2 is a task of planning and problem solving that can be used to investigate non-emotional decision making. Success on this task is impaired in mania and depression. Manic patients who tried the task had difficulty with even the easy levels, which could be due to difficulty with impulsivity and distractibility. As the levels get harder, their accuracy further decreases, and their responses become more impulsive [58]. Their responses are disinhibited. The impairment seen in mania on the cold decision-making task is a limited example, but it evokes the disinhibited and impulsive behaviour often seen during manic episodes: for example, unreserved spending and shopping sprees, promiscuity, gambling, reckless driving. The decrease in accuracy seen on the cold decision-making task is also observed in bipolar patients who are experiencing a depressed episode. These patients are especially bad at planning a strategy for tackling the task, and this planning ability worsens even more as the severity of depression increases [55]. These patients find it difficult to determine their next move and enact a plan; one can imagine how this impairment can grossly affect real-life decision making and strategizing.

In addition to the patterns of impaired decision making seen in mania and depression—increased errors and impulsivity, taking longer to make decisions, poor assessment of outcomes—depressed patients have difficulty learning from past mistakes. Part of the reason seems to be that they are especially vulnerable to negative feedback. During depressive episodes, they show catastrophic responses to their errors or misjudgements [59]. One way to think about this is that they are unable (or less able) to separate out each decision from the previous ones. This means that if they make an error on, say, question #3, their chance of failure on the next question dramatically increases compared with individuals who do not suffer from depression. In real life, this may manifest itself as giving up after a failed attempt, because they believe another failure is just around the corner. These perceived failures may result in them maintaining a negative outlook towards both themselves and external stimuli. If you recall, a leading therapy for depression is cognitive therapy, which emphasizes the importance of examining objective evidence for the sense of hopelessness and the negative beliefs that depressed individuals may hold. Another difficulty is that individuals suffering from depression cannot readily distinguish accurate negative feedback (e.g. being told you are wrong when you are, in fact, incorrect) from misleading feedback (e.g. being told you are wrong when you are in fact correct) [60]. This further affects their ability to use feedback to facilitate an improvement in performance. It may be that misleading feedback triggers a strong emotional response (for example, frustration or a sense of failure), which disrupts and influences the decision-making process.

* * *

What have we learned thus far? As we have seen, both the dorsolateral and orbitofrontal cortices are affected in the extreme emotional conditions of mania and depression. The activity in these areas of the brain is different from that of individuals without psychiatric diagnoses. Therefore, as predicted from the abnormalities seen in brain activation in the first part of this chapter, depressed and manic patients have difficulty with both hot and cold decision making. These difficulties have shown up in many studies, and are different from just saying that depressed or manic patients have poor overall cognition. In fact, these patients do not perform poorly on all tasks of cognitive function. However, their decision making is clearly affected, which in turn greatly affects their overall ability to function successfully in daily life.

Psychiatric patients have much to teach us about the brain's functionality in decision making, but they have both strengths and weaknesses as subjects for this kind of investigation. On the one hand, their conditions are well defined and there are, unfortunately, a large number of such patients. As a result, it is easier to find willing participants for a variety of investigations, and any insights have the potential to help a large population of patients, so research in this area has been strong. However, psychiatric conditions are notoriously complex, and until relatively recently have been treated as entirely non-physiological—as manifestations solely of the 'mind' or even the 'soul'. We are starting to learn more about the biological bases of these conditions, but the neurological basis is complex and there are also many environmental influences. It is unlikely that psychiatric disorders will ever be attributable to one physiological malfunction with a specific biological basis. After all, we have just seen how depressive and manic patients both have abnormal functionality in various areas of their brains (in addition to their orbitofrontal and dorsolateral cortices).

So although their symptoms reinforce our specific claims and help demonstrate the links of orbitofrontal with hot decisions and dorsolateral with cold decisions, it is not possible to make this attribution based solely on the difficulties seen in psychiatric patients. For additional clarity, we need to look elsewhere. The innovative brain scans discussed in Chapter 2 do play a role in making these attributions, but another source of insight is the much smaller but much more targeted set of investigations done with the input of neurologic patients—those whose brains have been altered by much more tangible and identifiable means.

Decision making in neurologically affected individuals

In contrast to psychiatric conditions, neurological conditions often have a more identifiable physiological basis. Therefore, it is possible to draw more clearly defined relationships between a particular injury to the brain and a particular cognitive deficit. Thus, we will examine a few types of neurological conditions involving damage to the orbitofrontal cortex and show how the dysfunction is relatively specific to hot decision making. Since damage to the orbitofrontal areas often includes parts of other nearby areas such as the ventromedial cortex, it may be more accurate to call some of these 'orbitofrontal-plus' injuries. The salient point, however, is that the orbitofrontal cortex is involved and these patients have difficulty with hot decision-making tasks. Importantly, these injuries do not affect the dorsolateral parts of the brain.

Research on patients with 'orbitofrontal-plus' lesions has supported the results gained from research into psychiatric patients. For example, when neurological patients with damage including the orbitofrontal-plus areas participate in the hot Cambridge Gambling Task that we have already described, they take longer to make their decisions, and also fail to choose the more favourable response [61]. This is reminiscent of the decision making seen in manic patients. Researchers have also noted that patients with ventromedial lesions place higher bets no matter the odds of winning; in other words, the orbitofrontal-plus areas seem to play an important role in making more conservative, safer—arguably wiser—decisions [62]. Patients with selective injury to the dorsolateral part of the prefrontal cortex do not show the same dysfunctional changes, which supports the conclusion that the dorsolateral cortex is not involved in emotionally laden decision making.

When patients with orbitofrontal-plus injury participate in a card selection task (called the Iowa Gambling Task) in which they can win or lose money, they also perform poorly—i.e. they fail to maximize their profits. In this task, four decks offer a variety of rewards and penalties: decks A and B provide high rewards and high penalties, while decks C and D provide low rewards and low penalties. Patients with orbitofrontal-plus injuries consistently choose the riskiest decks (decks A and B). In contrast, healthy individuals develop a preference for the decks with the highest overall profits (decks C and D). Patients with orbitofrontal-plus cortex injuries are not deterred by the increased risk of losing money, and do not seem to adapt their decisions based on the negative consequences they face (losing money and failing to maximize their winnings). The damage to their hot decision-making centres seems to impact their general ability to link their actions with their corresponding emotions [63].[32]

The evidence from these various studies has been used to support the Somatic Marker Hypothesis mentioned in Chapter 1. Researchers theorize that damage to the prefrontal areas may result in faulty 'somatic marking', which means that the patients are unable to link a somatic (body) state with consequences of their actions, so they continue to make poor decisions. The fact that these specific cognitive deficits are seen in various groups of patients who have suffered some abnormality to the same area of the brain—for either psychiatric or neurological reasons—supports the idea that the function of the orbitofrontal cortex is crucial for hot decision making. However, that is not the end of the investigation; there are at least two other neurological conditions that lend further credence to this notion.

Patients with extensive brain injury that includes *both* the orbitofrontal-plus and dorsal areas have a set of symptoms that are colloquially referred to as an 'acquired sociopathy' (or 'disinhibition syndrome'). These patients repeatedly engage in behaviours that have negative consequences for themselves, and make decisions that are neither personally advantageous nor socially acceptable. These changes in their decision making are not explained by changes in intellect, memory, language, attention, or perception. The 'acquired sociopathy' patients have a pattern of suboptimal decisions, and take longer to make their choices. An example of this syndrome can be seen in Phineas Gage. We suspect that the damage needed to bring about an 'acquired sociopathy' is more widespread because the more recent studies discussed above have shown that damage focused only within the orbitofrontal area results in prolonged deliberation on hot tasks, but not the sorts of widespread decision-making deficits seen in patients with 'acquired sociopathy'. For the diffuse deficits in decision making such as those seen in Phineas Gage to arise, patients need to have large frontal lesions that damage *both* the ventral/orbitofrontal and dorsal parts of the prefrontal cortex [31]. Put another way, the orbitofrontal area seems to be a necessary component for risky decision making seen in 'acquired sociopathy', but it is not sufficient alone to produce this syndrome. As an interesting aside, chronic amphetamine abusers with damage to the orbital regions of the prefrontal cortex show similar suboptimal decisions, and these suboptimal decisions correlate with years of abuse [61].

Our next neurological group includes those patients who suffer from damage to the frontal brain as a consequence of frontotemporal dementia (FTD). As we discussed above, FTD is a disease in which there is degeneration of the orbitofrontal cortex that contributes to a profound deterioration in personality and behaviour. FTD patients have changes in their personality: for example, apathy towards work, families, domestic responsibilities, an inability to organize a schedule, cravings for sweet foods and reduced satiety (and consequent weight gain), language difficulties, as well as other impairments of daily living [64]. The damage to the orbitofrontal cortex also greatly impacts such patients' ability to make emotionally charged decisions. They deliberate longer over hot decisions, and when they finally do decide, their decisions are risky and suboptimal [64]. Again, we can imagine the ways in which these difficulties might be expressed in everyday life.

The final neurological group we will look at includes patients who were fortunate enough to survive a very traumatic episode: a subarachnoid haemorrhage. Patients sometimes describe a subarachnoid haemorrhage as the sudden onset of the 'worst headache that they have ever had and could ever imagine'. This pain occurs when an artery coursing around the brain bursts, and one of the small spaces between the brain and the skull fills with blood. Eight to 12 per 100,000 people per year experience a subarachnoid haemorrhage, most commonly between the ages of 40 and 60 years. These subarachnoid haemorrhages can result from a ruptured blood vessel almost anywhere in the brain, but when the blood vessel is the anterior communicating artery (a common site for aneurysms), a large amount of damage to the orbitofrontal cortex can occur (see Figure 19). And as we might expect from the location of brain injury, these patients have difficulty with hot decisions: they place riskier bets, even after taking longer to deliberate [65]. These deficits are seen only on hot, emotional decision-making tasks. The neurologic patients behave in the same way as healthy volunteers on tasks of cold, rational decision making, which should not be surprising since the dorsolateral areas remain intact. Even though there are comparatively few of these patients, their unfortunate experience offers very

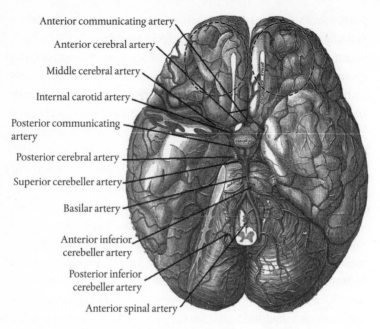

Anterior communicating artery

Anterior cerebral artery

Middle cerebral artery

Internal carotid artery

Posterior communicating artery

Posterior cerebral artery

Superior cerebeller artery

Basilar artery

Anterior inferior cerebeller artery

Posterior inferior cerebeller artery

Anterior spinal artery

FIGURE 19 Subarachnoid haemorrhage secondary to anterior communicating artery rupture will result in tissue damage, especially in the regions outlined by the dashed lines. These areas make up part of the orbitofrontal cortex. Image adapted from 20th US edition of *Gray's Anatomy of the Human Body*.

The Bodleian Libraries, The University of Oxford, 16544 d. 80

strong support for the connection between hot decision making and the orbitofrontal cortex. For the most part, these are otherwise healthy patients who undergo a single traumatic event and then show impairment on a very specific aspect of cognition.

What's next?

This chapter has dealt with a small selection of psychiatric and neurological patients and summarized some of the distinctive deficits that they show in highly regimented decision-making tasks. However, it is worth taking a moment to remember that although these deficits are measured in abstract ways, they manifest in nearly every facet of everyday life, and make life extremely difficult for these patients. Anecdotal stories about the experience of these patients should also help drive this point home. Each distinct deficit on a computerized battery of tests corresponds not only to a particular abnormality of brain function, but to life made more difficult and less enjoyable for thousands or even millions of patients and families. Until recently, the investigations into these deficits were just that—investigative—but as investigation and identification have become more widespread and precise, neuroscience is now able to at least partially treat some of these conditions. The evidence that these distinct but overlapping cases provide is crucial for helping researchers investigate different modes of improving—i.e. enhancing—decision making in these patient populations. In the case of these patients, the argument for doing everything possible to improve their cognitive capacity is clearly a strong one. Yet as we shall see in our final chapter, some of the same drugs that show promise for patients suffering from cognitive impairment also open up an ethical dilemma for healthy individuals who may seek not to alleviate cognitive deficits, but to improve intrinsic abilities. But first, in the next chapter we will investigate some of the treatments that already exist for the patients we have discussed thus far, and see how their decision-making abilities can improve with treatment.

4

INTERVENTIONS—DRUGS HIT THE PRESS

There are things that you can do today that, years ago, there was nothing [sic].
The [public] today needs to know that with MRI and the current medications
the view is good.   Teri Garr, actress

In the previous chapter, we looked at some of the medical reasons
why certain people have difficulties with decision making. It may
seem incredible that something as vague as 'bad decision making'
can be related to differences in function in specific parts of the brain,
but this seems to be true. In particular, we reviewed the deficits that
some psychiatric and neurological patients display when completing
computerized and other tasks, and we drew links between these difficulties and identifiable differences seen in the brain areas concerned
with emotional (hot) and rational (cold) decision making. For
instance, we learned that in individuals suffering from depression
and mania, the orbitofrontal (hot) and dorsolateral prefrontal (cold)
parts of the brain show abnormal activity. These individuals also
demonstrate impairments in emotional and non-emotional decision making, including slowed decision making, increased errors
and impulsivity, and a notable inability to assess outcomes properly.

Chapter 3 proposed some answers to the question of *why peo-*
ple make bad choices. Now we attempt to answer: *Can anything be*

done about it? We will explore a variety of cutting-edge treatments in use and under development today for psychiatric and neurological patients.[1] Each of these therapies has the potential to treat one or more disorders. This chapter is not intended to be a review of all possible treatments for the disorders already discussed, and we will focus our attention on treatments that can improve cognitive functioning, specifically the area of cognitive functioning that we have discussed throughout this book: decision making.

Brain surgery: treating cognitive and behavioural dysfunction with a scalpel

The first type of treatment we will focus on is the most dramatic, rapid, and invasive: surgery. By definition, surgical techniques attempt to improve the brain's function by physically altering it—a curious idea, particularly for problems as subtle as impaired decision making. It may seem like trying to repair your computer with a hacksaw.

Although it can achieve some remarkable feats, brain surgery has limits when it comes to cognitive enhancement. There are specific conditions and specific situations where a surgical intervention will help improve cognitive outcome, and times when it is absolutely necessary for survival. In general, however, surgery can only improve cognitive performance given a particular set of circumstances, and the improvement is relative to an impaired baseline. For that reason, surgery is not a primary treatment for psychiatric or neurological conditions, and is reserved for situations in which the benefit greatly outweighs the risk. It is usually a last resort.

Of the psychiatric and neurological disorders we have discussed thus far, surgical intervention is used most frequently to treat patients who have suffered a subarachnoid haemorrhage (SAH). Subarachnoid haemorrhage occurs when some of the space between the brain and the skull is filled with blood, usually after head trauma causes a blood vessel to burst. However, the haemorrhage can also be the result of an aneurysm. Aneurysms and haemorrhages are often misunderstood, but there is a difference between the two. A haemorrhage involves a broken blood vessel and bleeding into the surrounding tissue, whereas an aneurysm is actually the swelling of a blood vessel wall into a sort of balloon (called an out-pouching). Aneurysms are not necessarily harmful in and of themselves, but if they burst, then the haemorrhage that occurs is very dangerous. As a result, the primary reason for surgical treatment of a subarachnoid haemorrhage is to keep the patient alive, not improve their brain function. Patients with subarachnoid haemorrhage often require surgical intervention in order to prevent re-bleeding and further injury, or even death. Nevertheless, because SAH often results in damage to specific parts of the brain (as discussed in the previous chapter), the surgical treatments to alleviate the danger posed by the haemorrhage can also improve brain function in the affected area.

There are two surgical treatments currently available for treating the subarachnoid haemorrhage that results from a ruptured aneurysm: these are known as clipping and coiling. In the clipping method, patients undergo a craniotomy ('opening of the skull bones'), the vessels around the brain are exposed, and a clip is placed on the neck of an aneurysm in order to prevent blood from flowing into the vessel out-pouching (see Figure 20).[2] Think of this as clamping the neck of a balloon so that air can't get in or out. With a clip, the aneurysm still exists, but it is cut off from the rest of the circulatory system. Patients who undergo this treatment have fewer repeat episodes of bleeding in their brain. However, certain types of aneurysms and certain locations in the brain are difficult or impossible to clip.

Another type of surgical intervention developed at University of California, Los Angeles in the early 1990s is endovascular ('inside the blood vessel') coiling. In this procedure, the patient's skull remains intact, and no brain tissue need be disturbed. Instead, a small incision is made in the thigh, and a catheter is inserted into the femoral

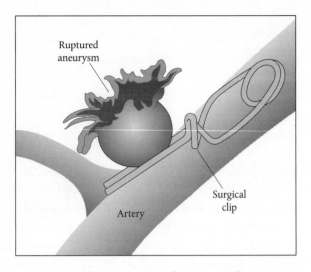

FIGURE 20   Clipping treatment for intracranial aneurysm.

artery and passed up through the aorta—the largest blood vessel in the body, which connects directly to the heart—into one of the arteries leading to the brain. Once in the appropriate brain vessel, the catheter is inserted into the aneurysm itself and fine metal coils are ejected into the out-pouching (see Figure 21). After the coils are inserted, the same components of blood that make a clot or scab after you accidentally cut yourself will help form a clot inside the aneurysm, and this lowers the risk of continued or repeated bleeding.

Put simply, clipping the aneurysm requires working from the outside inwards, while coiling works from the inside outwards. Endovascular coiling has a shorter recovery period than surgical clipping because the procedure itself is much less traumatic—it involves fewer incisions, less blood loss, and no cutting through bone. Unfortunately, there is a trade-off: although coiling definitely decreases the rate of re-bleeding compared with no treatment, the effect is not as robust as when clipping is used [66].

(A)   (B)

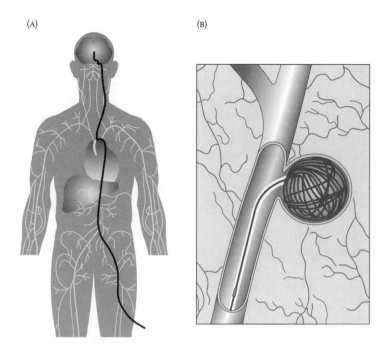

FIGURE 21 In endovascular coiling, a catheter is A) first passed through the femoral artery up to the brain and into the aneurysm, where B) coils are released into the aneurysm to aid the formation of a clot within the aneurysm itself.

Back to the main point of this chapter, though: can the available treatments improve cognitive functioning? When patients survive an SAH, cognitive impairment is a major obstacle during their rehabilitation. Do these surgical procedures improve cognitive function in these patients? The short answer is: yes, they help...but they do not cure. Despite neurological improvement after surgical treatment, the sufferers of subarachnoid haemorrhage continue to have difficulties with memory, executive functions (including decision making), and attention; some also exhibit personality changes.[3] The most important factor in determining outcome seems to be— unsurprisingly—the wait time before the intervention. Patients who had surgical intervention within three days of their haemorrhage make better-quality decisions later [67]. The *type* of surgery employed—clipping versus endovascular coiling—also seems to make some difference, but the results are not one-sided.

Patients who have undergone either surgical clipping *or* endovascular coiling have shown that their cognitive symptoms markedly improve over time. In other words, on average, over the long term, either kind of surgery is better than no surgery, even with the risks involved in the procedures. However, immediately following surgery, the story is different: both types of patients show some decline in cognitive functioning (presumably due to the trauma of the procedure), but patients who have an aneurysm clipped rather than coiled appear to have a slightly *greater* impairment [68]. This discrepancy can theoretically be explained because the clipping procedure itself is traumatic and involves opening the skull and possibly further disturbing brain tissue. Six months down the line (presumably after the patient has had time to heal from the invasive procedure), there is no notable difference in cognitive outcomes between the two types of procedure.

Unfortunately, surgery is far from an ideal tool for improving brain function: as we discussed above, it is invasive and usually only does one of two things: remove problematic features (such as a clot or bleed), or disrupt problematic brain activity (such as a seizure focus). The cognitive improvements achieved by surgery are real, and can make a dramatic, beneficial difference in the lives of patients...but these improvements are relative to what would happen with no treatment (i.e. death or more severe impairment). By its very nature, therefore, surgery has a somewhat limited utility in improving brain function, and we do not expect the currently available surgical techniques to play a cognitive-enhancing role. The most promising approach for treating individuals with cognitive impairment, and the one showing greatest potential for future advances in both impaired and healthy people, is pharmacology.

Acetylcholine: more is more

Patients with dementia are usually prescribed what is called an acetylcholine esterase inhibitor (AChE-I)—a medication that blocks the breakdown of the neurotransmitter acetylcholine, thereby increasing acetylcholine levels in the brain. Acetylcholine is thought to be involved in attention, memory, and other cognitive functions. In patients with dementia, levels of this brain molecule are low, and acetylcholine esterase inhibitors were developed in response to a long-standing theory that if we had a medication to increase the levels of acetylcholine, it would probably have positive effects on the brain's cognitive functioning. These medications are effective in treating some cognitive symptoms in Alzheimer's disease—particularly attention and concentration [69]—but they are not a total cure. In other words, acetylcholine esterase inhibitors do not improve dementia to the point that patients perform at pre-dementia levels. However, these medicines are still very useful and effective and are able to alleviate some symptoms, for example when patients show signs of inattention or disorientation. Acetylcholine esterase inhibitors are most helpful in mild and moderate stages of dementia while the neural circuitry retains a decent amount of residual function. These AChE-Is help patients function at a stable level for a longer period of time, which translates into more time at home (i.e. out of institutionalized care) and can increase patient independence while also decreasing medical costs. Another, more recent, study showed that these acetylcholine medications could be useful in the later stages of Alzheimer's as well [70]. The pharmaceutical industry is actively attempting to develop neuroprotective drugs that will halt the underlying disease process in Alzheimer's disease.

The evidence for cognitive improvement is clearer when these medications are given to healthy individuals. One study found that during a flight simulation task, pilots who took an AChE-I for one month were significantly better at manoeuvring during emergencies and landings [71]. This is evidence for cognitive enhancement in healthy individuals. Further evidence comes from another study, which found that the acetylcholine esterase inhibitor known as donepezil (Aricept) slightly enhanced memory function [72]. In general, however, the possible beneficial effects of acetylcholine esterase inhibitors are not considered worth the risk of side effects and possible interactions with other medications.

Methylphenidate: the first generation

Acetylcholine esterase inhibitors work on the premise that increasing the level of a specific neurotransmitter throughout the brain—in this case, acetylcholine—will have beneficial effects on cognitive function. The next medication we are going to discuss belongs to a different class of drugs altogether: the stimulants.[4] Prescription psychostimulants have historically been used to treat drowsiness and daytime fatigue, but the most commonly prescribed stimulant—methylphenidate,[5] also known as Ritalin—rather counterintuitively became popular as a treatment for attention deficit hyperactivity disorder (ADHD).[6] The period since 1990 has seen significant increases in production, consumption, and unfortunately also abuse of methylphenidate.[7] Abuse is an omnipresent threat because in addition to its therapeutic effects, methylphenidate has a collection of side effects that people sometimes find pleasurable.

Since methylphenidate is a stimulant medication, it has the potential to increase alertness. Methylphenidate increases levels of neurotransmitters (dopamine and noradrenaline) in parts of the brain where they are needed [73], and in this way has also been able to reduce impulsive behaviour and improve concentration in patients with ADHD. It may seem strange to treat a hyperactivity disorder with a stimulant, but the therapeutic outcome of this drug suggests that, despite the 'H' in its name, ADHD is perhaps better thought of as an inability to focus—of misdirected attention—rather than simply an increased level of physical activity. Methylphenidate does not only reduce the levels of physical activation in those with ADHD. Studies have shown that methylphenidate improves the low level of activity seen in some individuals, and it can also reduce abnormally high levels of baseline activity. In other words, the same drug can either suppress or encourage activity, depending on the patient's baseline state. The practical consequence of this is that methylphenidate is a fairly effective treatment for ADHD. In general, individuals with ADHD are better able to focus on tasks after taking methylphenidate.

This clinical picture is fairly clear, but how does the effect of methylphenidate manifest in the decision-making sphere? Methylphenidate helps to normalize the impulsive, risk-seeking behaviour seen in individuals with ADHD. Our research has shown that children with ADHD who are not taking medication routinely perform poorly on the Cambridge Gambling Task; they bet impulsively and do not adjust their bets in the same adaptive fashion that we observe in children without ADHD. However, some of these risky decision-making deficits resolved after taking methylphenidate [74]. In other words, patients taking methylphenidate bet more conservatively and in line with a successful strategy. While taking methylphenidate, the children with ADHD adjust their risky behaviour to be comparable with that of healthy children.

Given the excellent effects seen in improving the concentration and alertness of ADHD patients, recent research has diversified to see what effects—if any—methylphenidate can produce in individuals suffering from some of the psychiatric and neurological conditions we have discussed earlier in this book: depression, mania, dementia, etc.

Since the advent of traditional antidepressants (tricyclic antidepressants in the 1950s, and selective serotonin reuptake inhibitors such as Prozac in the 1980s),[8] interest has decreased in methylphenidate as a treatment option for uncomplicated depression. Initially, the effects of methylphenidate in depression had been mixed, with some studies claiming good effects on depressive symptoms, and others not showing an effect [75–77]. However, there are certain circumstances of patients developing depression who are extremely medically ill (for example, those patients in the intensive care unit, or terminally ill patients). These patients are not candidates for traditional antidepressant medications because of their delayed onset of action, side effects, and potential for interactions with other medications. Psychostimulants such as methylphenidate take effect within 36 hours and can provide another treatment option for severely ill, depressed patients such as these. A 2009 review of the available literature supported the view that methylphenidate is safe in these populations and that in the absence of data to indicate lack of efficacy, it should continue to be investigated [78]. In a very recent randomized, double-blind, placebo-controlled trial of methylphenidate in patients with limited life expectancy, researchers found that depression scores decreased in patients after treatment with methylphenidate. The methylphenidate was used for treatment of fatigue, which also significantly improved, and the improvement in depression scores may have reflected an improvement in their debilitating fatigue [79]. Studies investigating its use in bipolar disorder have been more positive, but are limited in number. Complementary treatment of bipolar disorder with methylphenidate results in improved depressive symptoms, although in one study the medication had to be stopped because of medication-induced hypomania ('mild mania') [80, 81]. Methylphenidate also augments the rate of improvement in elderly depressed patients [82]. Despite these positive results, methylphenidate is not primarily used to treat depression, and most research has focused on patients with neurological conditions. The effects of methylphenidate in neurological conditions—and specifically the effects on cognitive function—have been more promising.

Researchers have found that methylphenidate *does* improve decision making in certain neurological patients. For instance, it has been noted to improve decision making on the Iowa Gambling Task six months after subarachnoid haemorrhage injury [83], and has also been shown to ameliorate abnormal risk taking in frontotemporal dementia patients [84]. These patients' level of risk taking on gambling tasks was normalized with a single dose—just *one dose*—of methylphenidate, though the medication is given at regular intervals throughout the day to those who need it. Furthermore, methylphenidate seems to achieve these effects without causing the sorts of side effects normally seen in elderly patients, such as clinically significant changes in blood pressure and heart rate. These early results are very exciting, since they seem to show that even patients with severe physical brain injuries can benefit from certain medications.

These conclusions are supported by the experience of other patients who have suffered traumatic brain injury (TBI), who also seem to show cognitive improvement after taking methylphenidate. Some studies show improved memory and attention abilities [85–87], even if the patients do not receive other rehabilitative training. This means that even without specific coaching or training, these patients show improved cognitive functioning—a very rare outcome in TBI patients. Additionally, while administration of methylphenidate does not seem to make a difference in the overall *level* of recovery of cognitive function in patients with traumatic brain injury, the *rate* of recovery is more rapid for those who receive pharmacological enhancement [88]. In other words, methylphenidate alone doesn't help traumatic brain injury patients recover to a higher level of functionality than they would otherwise reach, but it does seem to help patients get there faster. This may seem like a minor point, but the rate of recovery is an important consideration for patient quality of life, particularly with rehab courses that can last for months or years. In addition, patients with traumatic brain injury who are given methylphenidate often have shorter intensive care unit stay times [89]. The implication is that methylphenidate can help patients be cognitively rehabilitated in a quicker, more efficient, and more economical time frame—a benefit in itself, despite the fact that the long-term degree of cognitive rehabilitation is unchanged [90].

Other studies suggest that methylphenidate could be used as an add-on therapy to counter cognitive decline in patients with progressive neurological illness such as tumours, Alzheimer's, or vascular dementia [91, 92].

The balance of evidence suggests that methylphenidate can produce notable, though not always dramatic, improvements in functioning in patients who suffer from a wide range of neurologic and psychiatric conditions. The interesting corollary to everything we have just discussed is that healthy individuals also show improvement in cognitive abilities when taking methylphenidate, and this has led to increasing reports of off-label misuse in both patients and healthy individuals. However, as you might expect, the reality of the research is more complicated than simply saying that methylphenidate has cognitive-enhancing effects.

Healthy individuals generally report feeling more alert, attentive, and energetic while taking methylphenidate. Studies have also shown positive effects on spatial working memory (working memory actively holds information in mind), and in planning of the sort used in cold decision making [93]. These positive effects on spatial memory and planning can be viewed as an example of *cognitive enhancement* as it is generally thought of by the public (i.e. improvement of cognitive ability beyond an individual's natural state). At minimum, methylphenidate seems to at least effect improvement in well-rested individuals, regardless of whether those individuals are patients (who improve towards their original, pre-illness baseline), or healthy (who improve beyond their normal baseline).

However, the outcome may not be as clear-cut for older adults, or in the case of sleep deprivation. On the one hand, recent personal discussion with researchers at the National Institute of Health revealed that the cognitive performance of sleep-deprived individuals was significantly better after they took methylphenidate as compared with a placebo [94]. On the other hand, an earlier study had concluded that methylphenidate seems to produce no cognitive-enhancing effect in sleep-deprived individuals [95]. And a third group of researchers has reported that healthy *elderly* individuals described a sense of increased alertness, energy, and proficiency despite not having a measurable improvement in cognitive function after taking methylphenidate [96]. In other words, these elderly patients *felt* more 'on top of their game' even if they did not actually perform any better. Taken together, all of these studies suggest that the enhancing effect of methylphenidate is real, but there might be an ideal age or dose range and state of rest within which the cognitive enhancement can occur.

Even with these caveats, this might seem like a clear case for the use of methylphenidate as a cognitive-enhancing drug, at least in certain patient populations under certain conditions. Unfortunately, methylphenidate, like any medication, has risks and benefits, and one must be aware of these risks and benefits when weighing its suitability for various individuals. In the case of methylphenidate, specifically, there is a strong abuse potential—the medication can be addictive.[9] Over time, if one's symptoms are not relieved by the same dose, or if one becomes used to a new baseline and tries to keep improving oneself, the temptation exists to increase the dose. At increased doses, however, the medication acts in ways other than intended, and can cause a mild euphoria that some individuals enjoy a little too much and pursue for its own sake. Other researchers have postulated that this abuse potential is complicated by the fact that people *feel* more alert—healthy people may feel as if the medication is enhancing their cognitive abilities even when it is not, in fact, doing so in any measurable way [95].

In addition to the abuse potential, there are other reasons why an individual should be hesitant to take (or prescribe) methylphenidate. It has been linked to heart attacks or sudden death in individuals with heart problems [97–99]. Long-term studies have also revealed that it has the potential to negatively impact children's growth [98]. For a medication with such potential for addiction, and such a wide base of paediatric patients, these are obviously serious drawbacks. They highlight one of the enduring truths of the medical profession: there are no miracle cures. Methylphenidate became a phenomenon, in part, because individuals—both parents and doctors—sought an easy and effective way to modify the behaviour and cognition of children with problems at home and school. Methylphenidate has been an important treatment for children with severe ADHD who otherwise might be excluded from or drop out of school. However, there is a risk of side effects (which were not as well known in the early days of methylphenidate's popularity). This consideration should be central in the development of any pharmacological treatment plan.

In response to these negative side effects, physicians and researchers have attempted to find another medication that might be used to achieve the same beneficial effects seen in patients who take methylphenidate, but without the same abuse potential. One such medication was approved by the Federal Drug Administration (FDA) in 1998 to treat the daytime drowsiness experienced by narcoleptics [100]. Its generic name is modafinil (also known as Provigil in the USA).[10]

Modafinil: the next generation

Modafinil is not a classic stimulant, nor does it have demonstrable abuse potential. The best term for it is 'wakefulness-promoting agent'. It is the medication that Nicole Kidman rummages for in the 2007 movie The Invasion, and which she takes to try to keep herself awake until she finds a cure for an alien virus. It is a medication that is FDA approved for use to treat the fatigue associated with narcolepsy, sleep apnoea, and shift-work sleep disorder. In addition to treatment of fatigue, modafinil has also been used 'off label' (i.e. without FDA approval) to treat a variety of other conditions such as attention deficit hyperactivity disorder [101], cocaine addiction [102], schizophrenia

[103, 104], Parkinson's disease [105], multiple sclerosis [106], and it is also used by many militaries to help keep personnel active for longer [107, 108]. The way in which modafinil achieves its effect is not entirely known.[11]

Different patients have different reactions to modafinil, and we cannot expect a single pill to magically help everyone. That said, it does seem to have beneficial effects for a wide range of patients. For instance, patients with schizophrenia are more flexible in their thought processes and planning, and also have some aspects of enhanced memory processes [104]. Patients with ADHD also seem to benefit.

A key study in our laboratory found that adults with ADHD who take modafinil show improved memory, among other things. They have improvements in cold decision making, with an increased ability to perform rational/non-emotional tasks [109]. This improved ability also manifests itself as the ability to stop doing something they are instructed not to do [109], such as inhibiting a particular behaviour. One could argue, perhaps, that these individuals experience an enhanced ability to focus on a particular behaviour and inhibit it when they are supposed to do so. In addition, these patients are more accurate. They take slightly longer to complete the planning and problem-solving tasks, but in the context of increased accuracy of answers, it may be that modafinil increases the ability to reflect on problems or decrease impulsiveness (i.e. improved decision making) [109]. The real-world implication is that these individuals may be able to perform the behaviours they want to while more easily inhibiting behaviours they do not want to perform. Since an inability to fully control one's actions is a key debilitating symptom of ADHD, improvement in this arena has the potential to significantly help improve patients' daily lives. ADHD is usually thought of as a childhood disease, but it frequently persists into adulthood. The results of this study also suggest that even though the cognitive benefits of medications like modafinil or methylphenidate are most often seen in younger populations, they are not limited to these young patients.

Other researchers have broadened our understanding of the effects of modafinil in various patient populations, although the results are not always as hoped. On the plus side, modafinil decreases the desire to gamble and normalizes risky (hot) decision making in highly impulsive, pathological gamblers [110]. But other patient populations—such as Huntington's disease patients—show either no effect or a deleterious effect from taking modafinil [111]. This is to be expected with any medication; there are always response differences in different groups of patients. The goal of further research is, of course, to find patient populations that can benefit from modafinil treatment and improve their quality of life, and also to quantify the longer-term effects of modafinil use. At present, our labs are, for instance, researching the effects of using modafinil in patients with traumatic brain injury.

Modafinil shows great promise for helping patients in psychiatric and neurological populations, and its use for these patients is complicated, though not especially controversial. The real controversy lies in the use of modafinil as a cognitive-enhancing medication for healthy individuals. Our lab has done some of the pioneering research in this area, usually investigating the short-term effects of limited doses. In these types of studies, healthy individuals or patients are usually given single doses of a medication, and then undergo computer testing, surveys, and/or imaging studies.

The clinical picture here is straightforward: modafinil has a positive effect on the cognitive function of healthy volunteers. Volunteers who are given a single dose of modafinil have improved results on both the hot and cold decision-making tasks that we have discussed in previous chapters; their decisions are more accurate and they deliberated for longer (i.e. were less impulsive or more reflective) [112]. This result indicates that they are trading the speediness of their response for the accuracy of their response, and this same speed–accuracy trade-off is observed in ADHD patients receiving pharmacological treatment. In addition to providing further evidence of improved decision making in healthy volunteers, another study also suggests that people who take modafinil find the tasks that they do more pleasurable after having taken the drug; in other words, modafinil may help people be more effective because tasks seem more enjoyable [113]. Other studies have found that memory abilities and attention are enhanced in certain tasks performed by young volunteers [114], but these results may not be evident in older volunteers [115]. On the other hand, older volunteers are better at tasks of spatial manipulation and mental flexibility after taking modafinil [115]. In addition, individuals with lower IQs tend to reveal a more notable enhancing effect when taking modafinil [116].

Modafinil's generalized cognitive-enhancing effect may have something to do with its primary function as a treatment for sleep deprivation. Sleep is, after all, probably the most dramatic cognitive enhancer we know of. We each know from personal experience that after a full night's sleep we are more 'on top of our game' and feel rested. Conversely, we also know that our sharpness decreases with decreased sleep. Unfortunately, most people do not get the optimal number of hours of sleep that they should, resulting in the all-too-well-known symptoms of sleep deprivation [117]: decreased alertness, decreased energy, difficulty processing information, mental lapses, decreased coordination and poorer reaction time, etc.[12]

The effects of sleep deprivation are well known to all of us. There is also a wealth of data to support what we intuitively know: sleep deprivation is detrimental to our academic and work performance. A good review on the subject provides these important points: 1) REM (which is when most of our dreams take place[13]) and non-REM sleep are both crucial for learning and memory, 2) students of different education levels suffer from poor sleep quality, which is due to a variety of factors, but this poor sleep quality contributes to 3) increased daytime sleepiness, impaired mood and behavioural changes, and cognitive deficits (particularly in areas such as attention, problem solving, decision making, etc.) [118]. This means that the all-nighters that students spend studying for exams are likely more harmful than beneficial. Lastly, when sleep is optimized, one can see improvement in cognitive function [118], i.e. the cognitive effects of poor sleep could be reversible. In the workplace, studies show that shift workers around the world have significantly more fatigue, poorer performance, loss of concentration, are more prone to having accidents and making errors, and are more likely to call in sick [119–121]. Moreover, the impact of sleep deprivation in the workplace is enormous; there is a loss of productivity at a high cost to the employer (estimated at $1,967 per employee annually in one study [122]). In fact, there is an entire new field within sleep medicine to address these effects of poor performance, lost productivity, and errors in the workplace [123]. Yet as we were preparing this book for publication, a news article noted that night-shift work is on the rise in both Britain and the United States [124]. It seems likely that the problem of widespread sleep deprivation is not going to disappear any time soon.

Sleep has become a luxury that many people do not or cannot make time for in our 24-hour society. Some professions expect their members to take a sort of perverse pride in working long hours—it is seen as a sign of dedication and capability (and, naturally, more billable hours per employee). Many others (shift workers, doctors, security guards, etc.) have to work through the night and thus prioritize work over sleep. To some extent, this is the price society has to pay for increased convenience and availability of services. However, when the people who are sleep deprived are in charge of other individuals' welfare, there are concerns that arise, and rightly so.

For instance, it is a simple fact that sleep-deprived physicians make more medical errors [125, 126], so we expect that decreasing physician fatigue would positively affect medical care. If sleep is not possible, medications like modafinil may help. Emergency room physicians who have taken modafinil have a marginally decreased number of errors on a task requiring continued attention, and also feel more alert [127]. Another study by researchers at Imperial College

London in collaboration with our group at the University of Cambridge found that doctors who took a single dose of modafinil after a long shift worked more efficiently, were less impulsive decision makers, and were more able to flexibly redirect their attention [128]. Anecdotally, colleagues have told us that once they finally get the chance to sleep, it can be more difficult to fall asleep after taking modafinil; however, these claims have been unsubstantiated in formal studies.

The military is another group that has to work long and continuous hours to achieve a mission. A number of countries—including the USA, the UK, and the Netherlands—have investigated modafinil's potential for maintaining the levels of wakefulness and cognitive function necessary for military success.[14] One group of researchers investigated the abilities of pilots who had taken prophylactic ('preventative') doses of modafinil and then stayed awake for 40 continuous hours. They discovered that the pilots who had taken modafinil reported less subjective tiredness [129]. From an objective standpoint, they did not evidence slowed brainwaves (which are typically seen when people are tired), and were able to perform like well-rested individuals on a number of simulator tasks known to be negatively impacted by sleep deprivation. The same group of researchers found that modafinil had similar effects on F-117 pilots who were tested after 37 hours without sleep [130].

Military studies, by their very nature, focus on a narrow range of subject characteristics and demographics, but there is strong evidence that modafinil is able to restore performance and alertness during times of sleep deprivation to at least near non-sleep-deprived levels in otherwise healthy persons. This claim has been substantiated by rigorous scientific research. In 2003, modafinil was approved by the United States Department of the Air Force as a 'Go Pill' for management of fatigue in certain aircrews [131]. The British Ministry of Defence has invested a considerable amount of capital in the 'smart pill' as well [132].

Taken together, one way to think about the general cognitive-enhancing effect of modafinil is this: those who are sleep deprived, those with lower IQs, individuals with psychiatric and learning difficulties have more to gain from cognitive enhancement, and modafinil positively affects these individuals. However, it may have something to offer a wider range of people, at least some of the time. Most of us are—at least occasionally—sleep deprived. There are times when we are not ideally rested, e.g. as new parents, when beginning work on a Monday morning, at the end of a long working week, after travelling. At these moments we are not able to perform at our best, even if we are not fatigued in a clinically relevant manner. In these instances, a pill such as modafinil might be beneficial.

Next steps

We have seen that medications such as modafinil and, to a lesser extent, methylphenidate, can have cognitive-enhancing effects on some neurological and psychiatric patient populations, and appear to be promising treatments for the deficits in decision making that these patients have. The intended, approved use of these medications to treat recognized disorders is a crucial one that can improve functional outcome, quality of life, and well-being for these patients. This use is relatively uncontroversial.

The controversy arises in other contexts, such as when these medications are used in paediatric populations. Paediatric patients present an unusually thorny ethical dilemma, because they combine two difficult qualities: children are not able to make decisions on their own behalf, and their ongoing development means that medications can have substantially different long-term effects from those seen in adults. Over and above these purely ethical issues, there is some concern about overprescription; in recent years, the rate of stimulant prescription has increased [133]. There are also troubling accounts of parents who seek to 'normalize' children's behaviour and cognition when it may already be within a perfectly normal range, and parents who simply seek to improve their children's behaviour or cognitive ability towards some imagined ideal standard. The effect of treating a healthy child whose brain is still developing is worrying, and the potential for abuse of a medication is sometimes overlooked. Many of these concerns apply to adult users of these medications as well. But the fact remains that despite the risks and dilemmas associated with these medications, the cognitive benefits are also real.

This trade-off between possible harm and reasonably confident potential for cognitive help is one of the factors that make cognitive-enhancing medication so ethically fraught. By enhancing cognition and decreasing risky decisions, these medications may be able to improve the cognitive processes of healthy individuals in everyday circumstances. If so, should they be used in this manner? Put another way, what is a medication ultimately *for*? *Would the average person have anything to gain*—even if it is simply preventing cognitive lapses as they become fatigued—*by taking a medication such as modafinil?* If the answer to these questions is 'yes', or even if enough people think that it is 'yes', then it opens up a whole set of ethical dilemmas, as we will explore in our final chapter.

5

PROFESSOR'S LITTLE HELPER— THE ETHICS OF ENHANCED COGNITION[1]

We are prone to thinking of drug abuse in terms of the male population and illicit drugs such as heroin, cocaine, and marijuana. It may surprise you to learn that a greater problem exists with millions of [people] dependent on legal prescription drugs.　　Robert Mendelsohn, American paediatrician

The 'quest for the smart pill' is a medical and sociological fact. For as long as history has been recorded, people have sought substances to boost their mental powers, longevity, and energy levels. As written in *The Economist*:

> Leaves, roots and fruit have been chewed, brewed and smoked in a quest to expand the mind. That search continues today, with the difference only that the shamans work in pharmaceutical laboratories rather than forests [134].

The key question today is whether we as a society will know what to do with one once it is identified [135], and whether its use would benefit society as a whole.

This chapter is about an important—yet misunderstood—neuroethical issue. It is our attempt to instigate discussion about the risks and benefits of cognitive-enhancing medications, because these questions are, primarily, public ones. When considering the use of these drugs in a healthy population, the role of the 'medical professional' changes considerably—the issue is no longer one of weighing medical risk versus medical benefit. Widespread use of cognitive-enhancing medication is primarily a social question, and it depends on proper and widespread understanding of the risks involved [136].[2]

It is not our place to supply the answers. Like those reading the book we are members of society and it is for all of us to decide the best outcome for our future. However, we do have experience with these medications and the relevant research, and we believe that decisions that affect the public well-being should be made on the basis of the best knowledge available. We want readers to be able to discuss these issues, and come to their own informed opinions on the increasing lifestyle use of cognitive-enhancing medications based on what they read, hear in the news, and discuss with peers.

In Chapter 4, we learned that medications that enhance cognition do exist. In fact, some of them have existed for a long time; as a class of medications, they are known as stimulants, and are illegal in the United States without a prescription.[3] Despite their beneficial cognitive effects, these medications can be extremely habit forming. In the previous chapter, we also revealed that some of these medications might have useful clinical applications to help to make patients and healthy individuals perform better: they appear to improve decision making, attention, memory, and various other cognitive functions.

The benefits that a healthy, normal individual might derive from these drugs may be different from the benefits that a patient receives, but both types of user seem to improve their ability to better control their behaviours and responses, focus attention, and manipulate information. 'Drug' may not be a nasty, four-letter word any more. Modafinil is being used with increasing regularity; the company that developed it sells hundreds of millions of dollars worth of the drug each year, and many ethicists are becoming concerned over this use. The realm of ethics inevitably takes us into subjective territory, but there are some basic questions on which we believe there is broad consensus.

It seems that the first important question to ask is about the role of medication. Should medications simply aim to improve a quantifiable physical malady (e.g. cure an infection, kill a parasite), or should we accept that there is an ethical use for drugs that simply aim to improve patients' quality of life? The list of medications that improve quality of life without curing an ailment is not insignificant: it would include everything from antidepressants to aspirin (not to mention Viagra). The vast majority of individuals would probably agree that yes, 'lifestyle' cognitive-enhancing drugs should exist, at least for adults who require them for memory and concentration problems caused by neuropsychiatric disorders or brain injury.

These sorts of lifestyle cognitive-enhancing medications have been prescribed for patients with brain injury, dementia, schizophrenia, and many other disorders for years now. We briefly discussed acetylcholine esterase inhibitors in the previous chapter. This class of medications does not return a patient with Alzheimer's disease to pre-illness functioning, but they are able to provide symptomatic improvement. Although it may seem trite, some improvement is better than none. Besides the benefit to the patient in terms of cognitive function and quality of life, this symptomatic improvement also removes some of the burden from caregivers and family. Such considerations have broad social significance in an era of rapidly aging populations in the USA, the UK, and elsewhere, and the medical costs that these populations will incur.

To give the reader some idea of the impact that a cognitive-enhancing medication can have, it has been estimated for the British population that if Alzheimer's dementia patients could be cognitively enhanced by *only 1 per cent*, the predicted increase in care costs over the next two decades (rising to £17 billion, ~1 per cent of GDP) would be all but cancelled out [137]. Age is a risk factor in Alzheimer's disease and currently, individuals in the UK are living on average to 75 (men) or 81 (women) years of age. The United States is expected to have similar demographic shifts in coming decades, but on a much larger scale. Cognitive enhancement is not simply an abstract ethical issue; it is an issue with huge, and growing, financial significance. In the elderly population, cognitive enhancement can be thought of as simply helping patients take care of themselves for longer than they might otherwise be able.

The use of these medications in the paediatric patient population is more controversial. Should medications that enhance cognitive function be prescribed and available for use in younger individuals? The diagnosis of childhood disorders such as ADHD has skyrocketed in recent years. Since the 1970s, stimulant medications that aim to improve concentration and alertness have been prescribed for children suffering from ADHD, and, as we saw in the last chapter, they seem to work well. Their cognitive-enhancing effects improve performance in school and normalize interactions with other children. However, many parents and individuals are concerned about the long-term effects of using such medications, citing possible growth stunting and cardiac risk [98]. Can people reasonably accept a risk of side effects for the possible benefits of cognitive improvements seen with medication? How long should such patients take the medication? And in the case of children, who makes these decisions? What level of academic or social difficulty must a child have before the risks of medication are acceptable?

The prognosis for children with severe ADHD is poor if they are not treated effectively. They have poorer educational experiences, higher dropout rates, and other problems including increased accidents. For this reason, the National Institute for Health and Clinical Excellence (in the UK) has approved methylphenidate for the treatment of moderate to severe ADHD within the context of psychosocial therapy. The questions above assume, of course, that childhood disorders can be reliably diagnosed. As we mentioned in the previous chapter, there is a legitimate concern about over-diagnosis and medicating 'normal' childhood activity levels and behaviour.

As you can see, the questions that accompany the use of cognitive-enhancing medications are quite complex, and we have already departed from the realm of broad consensus. But thus far we have only discussed the ethics of medical or psychiatric *patients* taking these medications. Whatever consensus there is about the ethicality of making new treatments available for cognitively impaired patients, it fragments immediately upon discussion of healthy individuals just looking for a pill to make themselves smarter or more alert.

The first complication probably arises from social norms. We recently stumbled upon an interesting and relevant passage in a highly entertaining book by Bill Bryson entitled *I'm a Stranger Here Myself* [138]. The author remarked upon a lecture that compared how companies market healthcare products in the United States and Britain. He noted that the same healthcare-related product is advertised differently in the two countries. For instance, in the USA, a given pill—such as an over-the-counter medication to combat flu symptoms—would be sold as a magic cure that could guarantee total relief. In the UK, however, the medication would promise nothing more than feeling a tiny bit better. The gist, as Bryson explained, was that "the British don't expect over-the-counter drugs to change their lives, whereas we Americans will settle for nothing less…people in [the USA] expect to feel more or less perfect all the time." Think about that last bit for another second: *more or less perfect all the time*. Wouldn't that be nice? But what would it mean, exactly? To be able to function on limited sleep, focus for a longer period of time, improve memory and mental functions, maybe learn a new language, spend less time rereading things…to be able to improve ourselves.[4]

In the previous chapter, we left the reader with a question: would the average person have anything to gain by taking a medication that potentially enhances cognition? We have discussed the range of benefits and the probable risks. Now take a moment to think about two closely related corollary questions, the ones at the heart of this issue: 1) *Would you take such a medication if it were available?* and 2) *Would you welcome a society where other people did so?*

Let us explore some of the reasons why someone might answer 'no' to these all-important questions.

It's unnatural

Perhaps you say no because you believe that human ingenuity is something that seems diminished by the help of an enhancing substance. Like steroids in sports, it would cheapen any accomplishments. This argument has intuitive appeal to many. However, the line between 'natural' and 'unnatural' cognition is not at all clear-cut.

Thanks to human accomplishment and innovation over thousands of years, we have developed certain luxuries that have allowed us to enhance our brains. For instance, written language is a huge cognitive enhancer that has been around for a very small segment of human evolutionary history, and that until very recently has been limited to a minority of the population (in certain countries this is still the case today). Yet it has been socially transformative, by enabling much more complex and nuanced thought. Written language facilitates learning and puts a huge amount of reference material within the reach of individuals.

The computer, and more specifically the Internet, is a radical step further along that path. With the worldwide web at our fingertips, an enormous amount of information is within reach in seconds. Physicians, for instance, already use smartphones to look up medication doses, rare disease entities, and recent primary literature in order to better guide their treatment plans and advise their patients. Nowadays, there's an app for pretty much anything.[5] The Internet essentially acts as an external hard drive for the brain and, in that sense, allows physicians to improve their cognitive capacity. Instant access to reliable external data is a cognitive enhancer. Some may think, 'Wait; easy reference means I don't rely on memory so much and can expend more energy on other things.' If so, isn't that a sort of weakening of the brain? For instance, anyone reading this book will certainly have noticed that over the past decade it has become unnecessary to remember phone numbers. Nowadays, phone numbers are nearly always stored in our mobile. Is this an enhancement or a degradation of our cognition?

This brings us to an important point: cognitive-enhancing drugs improve a patient's ability to *perform certain mental tasks more effectively and efficiently*. This is not quite the same thing as being 'smarter'. The effect of these drugs is on performance. Therefore, a development that allows someone to perform more effectively (e.g. the doctor's iPad with medication doses and interactions cross-referenced) is an enhancer, even if we acknowledge that the individual doctor may not have such a sharp memory for drug names as was previously the case. It is important to keep this distinction in mind throughout any discussion of cognitive-enhancing drugs, because the question of what it means to be 'smart' is, of course, a complex one in its own right.

It may be helpful to think along the following lines: cognitive performance in different areas is a component of intelligence, but it is not the same thing as being smart. Cognitive performance is necessary, but not sufficient, for intelligence. After all, Dustin Hoffman's character in *Rain Man* (to cite one famous example) was very good at certain cognitive tasks, but only a sophist would call him generally 'smart'. So when we talk about cognitive-enhancing drugs improving cognitive performance, remember that they are playing a role more like an iPad or a Rolodex than a generalized thinking cap. They may help people do certain things more effectively, but the synthesis of this information is the true seat of intelligence.

With that in mind, we should reconsider the central ethical question at stake here: are cognitive enhancers ethical when taken by healthy patients? Medication and technology are both cognitive enhancers because they help us do more, and more effectively. We may feel that these improvements are not worth the cost, or the dependency, but it is important to recognize the question we're answering. Cognitive-enhancing drugs are *not* designed to make your life easier per se (though they may often be pitched that way). They are designed to improve (increase) your functionality and output. To put it in a slightly less pejorative way, they are designed to help you do more in a given time, and to do it more accurately. The fact of the matter is that we're seeking cognitive enhancement all the time. Technology just seems like a different avenue to the same goal. The difference might be that technological aids such as a computer are external and can be turned off or removed.

If that's true, then what about nutrition, exercise, sleep—are all of those so different? As we mentioned earlier, sleep is a huge enhancer of brain function, but no one would think of getting a good night's sleep before an exam as cheating. Then what about a student with insomnia? Is that student just naturally doomed to constant suboptimal performance due to an inability to sleep? If nutrition, exercise and sleep are steps taken towards making your body and mind function more effectively, then how is that different from taking a pill? Why is, say, vitamin D good but methylphenidate is bad? Are the effort and self-sacrifice involved in those 'traditional' methods of self-improvement an end in themselves? Is easy improvement inherently bad? If so, why? Might that opinion be a vestigial remnant from a time when easy improvement wasn't possible?

The issue is further complicated by the uncomfortable reality that cognitive-enhancing drugs are not a new and strange class of substance. If Starbucks is any indication, the issue of whether or not cognitive-enhancing drugs are socially acceptable has already been settled. The average reader—and the sleepy-eyed students we mentioned in our preface—probably would not think twice about ordering a vanilla latte or double espresso, and yet caffeine is also a cognitive-enhancing drug. This is not just academic pedantry;

caffeine increases alertness, decreases reaction times and improves cognitive function in people who are fatigued, in a way similar to other medications we have discussed [139–143]. Indeed, that effect is one of the main reasons for widespread coffee—and, to an extent, tea—drinking in societies where many adults are perpetually sleep deprived.[6] The common sentiment that 'I can't function properly before I've had my coffee' will certainly be familiar to you, even if it is not your personal view. Nicotine has similar effects, and although it is regulated, taxed, and demonized in both the UK and the USA, it is not illegal. In fact, Paul Newhouse and colleagues recently reported that people with mild cognitive impairment who wore a nicotine patch for six months performed better on tasks of mental processing and memory [144].[7] Clearly, the category of 'cognitive-enhancing drug' is not as exotic as it might seem at first.

Perhaps it is only a matter of time before we can go to the corner coffee shop and order a caramel macchiato with a shot of 'smart drug'. Maybe two shots. As of 2012, more than 21 million people in the UK are aged 50 and over (the age when people most frequently start to notice cognitive slowing); should these people be allowed to pop a pill in order to get through their day more successfully? Or simply maintain their performance in the face of fatigue? If not, who decides to ban a particular drug, and who enforces the decision? Many of the people who are suspicious about the use of such drugs are also very suspicious about government interference with individuals' rights.

Popularity is not the same as ethical justification, but in a revealing poll in the journal Nature, 80 per cent of readers felt that healthy adults should be allowed to take an enhancing medication if they chose to do so [145]. The results of this informal poll of 1,400 individuals representing sixty countries include some statistics that should influence the debate. One in five respondents admitted to having used a cognitive enhancer—methylphenidate (Ritalin), modafinil (Provigil), or other—to stimulate brain function (i.e. for a non-medical reason). Of those who have used such drugs, 62 per cent opted for methylphenidate, 44 per cent had tried modafinil, and 15 per cent had utilized a different enhancing medication [145]. As the percentages indicate, some respondents have actually tried more than one type of cognitive-enhancing medication. Reasons given for use of enhancing drugs included attempts to improve concentration and focus, as well as to fight jet lag.

Should students who need to stay up late to prepare for an exam be forbidden from taking a pill to perk themselves up? What would the purpose of such a prohibition be? Students already study all night with coffee or energy drinks such as Red Bull an arm's length away, after all. The fact is, non-prescription use of prescription stimulants such as methylphenidate is on the rise in high school, and on college and university campuses [146, 147].

Our species is driven to improve itself. Whether it is by exercising, achieving adequate nutrition or sleep, reading, wearing eyeglasses, using the Internet, obtaining safe housing, wearing warm clothes, etc., we are improving ourselves in unnatural ways. Modern urban and even rural life is profoundly unnatural in any evolutionary sense of the word—we live in environments and have access to resources that were unimaginable even a century ago, let alone a millennium. Medical advances are by definition unnatural: prenatal care has allowed more babies than is 'natural' to be carried to term; antibiotics have allowed people to survive infections from which they would otherwise have perished; corrective eye surgery has allowed people who would otherwise have gone blind to see again. At the neurological level, nearly every condition of our modern life—including medicine, education, and nutrition—can alter brain connections and function, and move it away from the 'natural' state [148–151]. In addition, these advances and resources are not equitably and evenly distributed even *within* countries, let alone between them. What, then, does it mean to promote 'natural' cognition as an ideal?

Not to disparage sensitivity to our natural condition, but from a medical and functional perspective, 'naturalness' is wildly overrated. After all, as Thomas Hobbes noted in *Leviathan* in 1651, the *natural condition* of mankind is one with no industry, agriculture, navigation, construction, timekeeping, art, society, or literature; a state of constant conflict and violent death, and of life "solitary, poor, nasty, brutish, and short".[8] He further argued that the social contract is an unnatural imposition to try to alleviate the natural state of mankind. We should be careful not to use 'natural' as a synonym for 'all the advantages I personally have, but nothing more'.

So it seems that singling out these drugs for being an unnatural attempt to improve cognitive function is really a confused argument. Rather, many of the objections to cognitive-enhancing medications being unnatural are really arguments that such medications are inequitable for one or another reason. This is a much stronger and more persuasive line of argument against such medications, as we will see below.

'It's not fair!'

There are two intertwined issues at stake when we discuss the fairness of using cognitive-enhancing medications for achievement. The first is whether such use is ever permissible, and the second is whether the inevitable inequality of access to such drugs creates an unfair environment for those who do *not* use them.

As for the first point, although it is a subjective issue, there is something that most people find inherently disturbing about 'doping' to achieve. Most would say it cheapens the accomplishment. The obvious analogy is seen in sports, where doping has been prohibited (and widely seen as unacceptable) for many years (though many fans profess not to care what professional athletes do to their own bodies). In fact, a recent study from researchers at University of Pennsylvania investigated attitudes towards cheating in either the academic or athletic realm. Of the 1,200 male students surveyed, a larger number of participants believed that an athlete who used anabolic steroids was more of a cheater than a student who used Adderall (a stimulant) to help him on his midterm exams [152] (though a survey of professional athletes might give a very different result!). Notably, the surveyed participants were more likely to have used prescription stimulants within the last year than anabolic steroids at any point in their lives; they also felt that Adderall was more necessary for success.

Clever students who have been admitted to top academic institutions in the United States and United Kingdom confess to using these medications to give themselves a little boost.[9] Does this fall outside the usual attempts by students to improve themselves by every possible means? Is it actually cheating? If so, how? The pills, after all, do not grant information or abilities; they *may* permit students to acquire them more effectively. Perhaps we will need to begin random drug testing before students are allowed to sit examinations. One survey estimated that between 7 per cent and 25 per cent of students have used prescription stimulants (whether their own or someone else's prescription) to give themselves a perceived edge [153].

Others argue that the concern is overblown, since intelligence is defined by multiple factors and, therefore, these medications are unlikely to give the type of overall boost that people seek. As we discussed above, even though these medications provide a measurable improvement in specific cognitive functions, it is still quite unclear whether they provide a boost or improve actual learning capability in otherwise healthy individuals when used long term. Nevertheless, if these medications do improve learning potential, there are clear implications for the educational system as a whole.

The presence of a pill-driven boost among some students could prevent a given testing measure from being able to accurately determine an individual's baseline competence, and would skew the results for the student body as a whole. This gets to the second 'fairness' dilemma mentioned above: inevitable inequality of access. These drugs are not free or universally available, nor will every student want to take them even if they were. Those who do not join in such cognitive extravagance might be left behind in the struggle for top-notch academic performance, and the gap between successful and unsuccessful widened even more. And now that standardized tests are playing an ever more prominent role in admissions and hiring decisions, the ability to score better on such exams should not be dismissed simply because it is different from being broadly 'more intelligent'. This temptation towards purely lifestyle-driven use of cognitive-enhancing drugs by the student population is perhaps not surprising since the Academy of Medical Sciences 2008 report on brain science, addiction, and drugs states that "small percentage increments in performance can lead to significant improvements in functional outcome". For instance, it is conceivable that a 10 per cent improvement in memory score could lead to an improvement in an A-level grade or degree class [154].

This controversy seems to map very closely onto well-known debates about the value of hard work and the reprehensibility of cheating. But there are important differences. If these medications were able to increase the overall learning potential of the population, then perhaps there exists the real opportunity for society-wide improvement. If that's the case, cognitive enhancement is quite different from the doping that is disdained in sports; it's closer to something like a nutrition initiative or a universal literacy programme that aims to give students an additional tool to help with their learning and achievement. In this case, rather than prohibition, there would need to be a concerted effort to ensure that everyone who wanted these medications had access to them. The use of cognitive-enhancing drugs would be akin to getting a good night's sleep—common-sense steps that responsible students should take to maximize their learning opportunities.

If you say that these medications are not fair, then what is fair—caffeine; nicotine; a beta-blocker medication to treat nervousness during public speaking; paid tutoring for admissions or exams (also not available to everyone)? The line between fair and unfair gets noticeably fuzzier the closer one looks. The issues at stake in the medically influenced learning arena are more complex, if only because they affect nearly every individual (or at least every family with children). A simple 'I know fair when I see it' argument is not enough, particularly when we are talking about setting public policy for both students and adults.

'But everyone else is doing it'

A formal published survey has estimated that 5–16 per cent of US students currently use cognitive enhancers, and an anonymous survey of 1,000 students at Cambridge University in England found that approximately 1 in 10 students admitted to taking a prescription medication such as methylphenidate without a prescription to help them work [155]. Anecdotally, the students say that the competition is too extreme, and the pressure to achieve is too much to conquer without a little help. The drive for success and achievement is a strong one, perhaps even stronger than the drive to be beautiful or athletic.

Consider: would you allow your elementary school child to give himself or herself a little boost? How about in secondary school? And if *everyone* else in their class was doing it and competing for the same spots at university—what then? Frequently, coercion becomes an issue. That is, students feel pressure to take smart drugs because they know other students who are taking them. In the *Nature* survey discussed above, 33 per cent of respondents said that they would feel pressure to give their children drugs if they knew other children at school were taking them. Popular is not the same as ethical, but it is a strong driving force that can shape behaviour in the absence (or even the presence) of ethical clarity.

'It's illegal, isn't it?'

Drug abuse is illegal. Doping in sport is illegal. Prescribed drugs are legal and, more often than not, are also beneficial. We, of course, do not support anyone obtaining medications illegally or outside consultation with their physician, but cognitive enhancement achieved through the use of a prescription drug is at least potentially 'legal'. Unfortunately, patients and parents who want to make an informed decision about the use of cognitive-enhancing drugs will not be able to rely on a simple metric of legal versus illegal. The relevant laws can, and do, change. There are different jurisdictions at the local and nationwide levels. Even when the laws are well known, it is quite common to hear about judgments being overturned or laws being repealed, often by a split decision. In other words, *professional legal interpreters* disagree about whether something is legal or not. Legality is probably the most clear-cut issue at stake in this debate, and yet it is not intrinsically clear at all. One of the reasons we feel this debate is so crucial is because the legal framework for the use of cognitive-enhancing drugs will be established, at least in part, due to the input and votes of informed citizens. In order to shape our opinions about legality, we must address *ethical* versus *unethical*, and *moral* versus *immoral* issues instead.

As one author wrote: "cognitive-enhancing drugs require relatively little effort, are invasive, and for the time being are not equitably distributed, but none of these provides reasonable grounds for prohibition" [156]. In a free society, the onus should be on a regulatory body seeking to ban a substance to prove that it is imperative to ban it; otherwise people should be able to make their own choices, correct? To put the question in more general terms: what is the purpose of making a substance illegal?

One of the most compelling reasons for proposing a ban on cognitive-enhancing medications is because of a fear of side effects. This is quite a reasonable concern. Any medication can have side effects, and these side effects are one of the biggest deterrents from taking a medication. Although modafinil has minimal side effects in the short term, the long-term side effects in healthy people are largely unknown as there are as yet no long-term studies.[10]

On the face of it, this seems a compelling argument. It is perhaps a persuasive argument to a parent, and could be an excellent reason to make sure your child does not take methylphenidate. However, we would argue that it should not be a persuasive argument to a legislator. After all, many substances with more dubious beneficial effects and more clearly known harmful side effects—tobacco and alcohol being among the most common, along with any number of 'alternative medical treatments'—are legally available, and widely used, simply because many people like them. If government's role is to ban every substance with potentially harmful side effects, there will be scant resources left.[11]

As we have argued above, the issues being considered with respect to current cognitive-enhancing drugs have mostly already been resolved in the public arena, even though many people do not think of them as being related. For instance, it is well known that caffeine is frequently used to increase an individual's productivity. It is less well known that caffeine has side effects similar to those experienced by people who have taken modafinil. Caffeine is widely available, effective, and in common use; however, at the dose required for its transient wakefulness-promoting effects (roughly 600 mg), side effects including tremor, anxiety, and nausea are common [128]. Our point is not that caffeine and modafinil are the same; modafinil is much more potent and its effects on humans are not well understood. Our point is simply that this debate involves issues already familiar to most patients and physicians.

One legitimately frightening issue, however, is that many of the students using methylphenidate and modafinil are not getting the medicines from their physicians. They are turning to other, more dangerous methods, such us purchasing medications over the Internet,[12] using a friend's prescription, and some even admit to crossing international borders to get the medications in countries where prescriptions are not necessary. Even more upsetting is that millions of people are estimated to have misused these medications, with addiction (in the case of stimulants) an omnipresent possibility. If we compare sales figures with prescription figures, it is clear that people are using modafinil without prescriptions. The dangers of drug misuse are largely separate from those of ethics—patients with unknown drugs in their systems are difficult to diagnose and treat because of unexpected side effects and drug interactions. If these drugs are to be used more widely, it is imperative that this is done within the structure of professional medical care.

An enhanced society

What are the reasons for the increasing lifestyle use of these smart drugs by healthy people? Research suggests that the two key reasons for this are to 1) gain a competitive edge, and 2) make routine or tedious tasks more pleasurable [113]. So what will be the next steps in the social debate over cognitive-enhancing medications? Currently, non-prescription use is not monitored—should it be? How can it be? How much would it cost to do so, and is the cost worth it? Does society even have a place in this discussion, or do people have the right to do to their bodies as they wish, even if this could potentially be harmful? Some people argue for putting tight regulations around these medications and banning them from use in healthy individuals, citing the fact that the medications currently on the market are potentially dangerous, unnecessary, and self-indulgent, and therefore bad.[13]

However, no one puts legal limits on the number of shots of espresso one can have in a 24-hour period—that would be ridiculous. If a medication were known to be comparatively safe—safer even than caffeine—could society rightly deny it from everyone except those who are cognitively impaired? At that point, maybe it would be beneficial to all if we put the smart drugs straight into the water, like fluoride. Many people would find that idea unsettling or repulsive, but if such drugs improve cognitive performance and societal productivity, how would it be different from, say, mandating nutritional standards for school lunches? Or encouraging vaccinations? Or setting school curricula? There is, of course, quite a range of possibilities between outlawing a substance and putting it in the drinking water.

Moreover, some healthy individuals clearly stand to benefit society *more* when they use these medications: military personnel are probably the prime example and the least controversial one since success in their missions usually has direct personal benefits as well as societal ones. Most would agree that soldiers have a right to every advantage—technological, physical, and cognitive—and that aiding them is in our best interest as a society. Where does one draw the line between who should and who should not receive cognitive-enhancing and wakefulness-promoting medications? How about airline pilots or surgeons? Nuclear plant technicians? Air traffic controllers? School bus drivers? Should CEOs who often need to adjust to time changes be allowed to give themselves a little boost? Being on top of their game is good for the company, and thus good for society, yes? Some scientists and professors have confessed to using the medication to help them battle jet lag or cope with intellectual challenges. If their research leads to important scientific advances, does that make the cognitive enhancement acceptable? To put it another way: if professionals take these medications and gain better outcomes as a result, what would be the point of banning the drugs? Plenty of expensive, ineffective placebos are already on the market, some of them with potentially serious side effects of their own.

To come at the same issue from another, more controversial, direction: if such enhancement is possible, do we have the responsibility to *require* pilots, for example, to take cognitive-enhancing medications? After all, regulatory bodies require them to abstain from alcohol and get a certain amount of sleep. What happens the next time a plane crash is blamed on pilot error, inattention, or falling asleep in the cockpit? Are the risks of such drugs worth the increased risk of errors being made? Are they worth the risks to the people taking them?

What rights do we collectively have to demand peak performance from people in key positions?

One prominent neuroscience researcher has asked, "If we can boost our abilities to make up for the ones Mother Nature didn't give us, what is wrong with that?" [157] And what *is* wrong with that? Doping in sports is vilified for many reasons, but key among them is the fact that the *competition* is itself the critical metric, and an unfair competition is essentially no competition at all. The doping negates the purpose of the sport. Apart from competitive admissions to universities and jobs, that metric does not really apply to everyday life. Even in exam settings, better group performance is not a bad thing per se. If every student aced their A-levels this year, that would make university admissions a nightmare, but it would not be a bad thing for the students themselves. Everyone doing better means everyone doing better, which is supposed to be the *point* of education, after all. Are we reaching a point in human history when we can begin to augment our minds, much like medicine and nutritional science have helped us augment our bodies and stave off death? Or is there something different about the mind, about cognitive functioning? Are we concerned that these drugs could change who we are as people?

In the course of conducting our research and writing this book, we have met many people who are willing to tell you exactly what is wrong with cognitive enhancement, and it can be summarized in the following way: the purpose of medicine is to heal the sick, not improve the healthy [158]. As we've argued above, we believe the reality is considerably more complicated, and that many common and accepted medical interventions (e.g. vaccines, prenatal counselling) do precisely that; they improve the healthy. Issues that have been raised in response to increased concern about cognitive-enhancing medications include the safety of such medications (side effects and long-term complications), the inequity of availability (given the cost, not everyone would have equal access to the medications), the risk of medication interactions (it introduces another possible variable into other medical treatments), peer pressure (if everyone else is doing it, wouldn't you *have* to as well in order to be competitive?), and a redefinition of sense of self (are you the same person you were before you were 'enhanced'?) [145].

Does whether it is 'right' or 'wrong' perhaps depend on the goal of the person taking the medication—the *mens rea* of traditional legal reasoning? In other words, is the exact same behaviour acceptable if done for purposes of wakefulness in order to help others (e.g. healthcare personnel) but not if done for exam preparation or out of the desire to be able to impress a client after an eight-hour flight? Or should people be allowed to do as they like so long as they are not harming anyone else with their decisions? If so, who gets to determine what 'harm' is (especially for children), and how much is too much to allow?

In general, it seems like one thing people do agree on is that if these medications are going to be around, then three things need to happen: 1) further research into the long-term risks and benefits of these drugs in healthy people, 2) formation of guidelines (at least) about who should and who should not be taking these cognitive enhancing drugs, and 3) education of professionals, teachers, students, and the public about the risks and benefits.

Further research

At this time, there are lots of things we do not know about cognitive-enhancing medications. For instance, we know little about real-world effects outside the controlled laboratory environment, with the exception of anecdotal stories and claims. Therefore, we need to investigate how these 'smart drugs' affect—if at all—real people in real-world situations. Another important research question is whether these medications are able to alter the way that people learn and assimilate information, or if they just act to give a boost in order to temporarily cram in more information. Is total knowledge increased, or perhaps the transient rate of knowledge accrual? What happens when someone who has been taking the drug suddenly stops? Additionally, most cognitive-enhancing medications seem to be relatively well tolerated, but what are the risks for addiction and abuse?

At the moment, there is also much we do not understand about the side effects of such medications, especially about the long-term effects on development. The risk of unexpected side effects is high, and may not be inconsequential. Most importantly, the significance of the patient's age is not well understood. For instance, is a child more at risk of certain side effects or at a higher likelihood of developing dependence than an adult, or vice versa? Might certain drugs have detrimental effects on a child's development? There is reason to suspect these risks are real, since children are usually more sensitive to any given medication, and their ongoing development means more opportunities for harm. However, future progress may offer promising avenues for making these drugs safer. As research into pharmacogenomics—that is, how genes affect your body's response to drugs—continues, it may be possible to customize medication choices to minimize side effects. In the future you may be able to determine which cognitive-enhancing drug is both safe and effective for you based on your genes.

Safety should be a priority, but scientific research is necessary to help define public policy. Any policy should attempt to incorporate evidence-based findings as they become available and more information is known about these medications and drugs.

Legislation

In taking steps towards making policies and guidelines, it is important to include relevant people. These people include those professionals who manufacture, dispense, prescribe, or even use cognitive-enhancing medications. In particular, physicians need to be aware of these medications, because physicians are, in large part, the gateway to these medications. Primary care physicians, neurologists, paediatricians, and psychiatrists probably prescribe these medications more often than other specialities. Given their large role in regulating these medications from the perspective of providing a prescription, it seems reasonable that the professional societies for physicians (for instance, the Royal College of Physicians or the American Medical Association) should provide guidelines and promote discussion on the ethics of prescribing cognitive enhancers. They should also provide guidelines about appropriate candidates for these medications.

This is not the first time a professional society would provide such guidelines. For instance, women undergoing in vitro fertilization are subject to limitations. Although it is not illegal to implant, say, thirty embryos, it is unethical to do so, and medical guidelines exist to guide doctors' decisions. They also exist for transplant recipients and cosmetic surgery. Professional societies are becoming more and more involved in the ethics of professional behaviour, perhaps in part because these are difficult issues for individual practitioners to address.

The academic community is also intimately involved in the repercussions of cognitive enhancers: educators, admissions committees, examiners. These professions will have to assess their stance on the matter, and how it affects the application and admission process— and then after admission, how it affects the examination process. They will have to discuss how they will ensure the integrity of their exams and student assessments. Similar discussions have occurred in the past in the context of standardized testing, as well as test taking by people with disabilities.

There are, of course, many more professional societies who should address guidelines for use of cognitive-enhancing medications: pilots, military, human resources, pharmacists, surgeons, to name a few. Many different professionals potentially stand to benefit from enhancement, though the value of this enhancement will likely be varied among professions [159]. However, another goal is also to ensure that individuals using these drugs are protected from harming themselves. For instance, many medications cannot be taken in combination because of dangerous interactions in the body. The point of channelling cognitive-enhancing medication use through the aegis of professional societies is to ensure that people who use these medications are as safe as possible.

The professional societies then need to cooperate with legislators to safely control these substances in a manner that will benefit both the individual and society. In our opinion, the government's role in all of this is to coordinate and *recommend*, to *guide* its citizens. It also ideally needs to continually modify recommendations and any legislation in order to incorporate new data, particularly as regards harmful effects.

There is a multitude of ways that this issue can be addressed. Some have proposed a laissez-faire approach (free-market free-for-all where those who want it and can get it are able to use it), while others have proposed that the government should make these medications available for all to use, and still others have advocated for strict regulatory legislation and structure, or outright prohibition. There are many options that fall somewhere in the middle of these extreme stances. The government may ultimately have to determine which of these cognitive-enhancing drugs are safe so that they can be marketed and people can obtain them safely, after consultation with their doctor, rather than purchasing them on the Internet. In any case, the focus should be on permitting the safe use of efficacious medications while minimizing harm.

Education

One of the most important roles in the discussion of these contentious issues is education. Not only the individuals taking and prescribing the medications, but also the public in general should be engaged in educational discussions about these medications. Importantly, this education needs to include the danger of obtaining these medications from unofficial sources, and the concern of these medications producing side effects or interacting with other drugs. We have insisted from the start that our intention is to inform a discussion about smart drugs—their risks, as well as their benefits.

This book is meant to portray both sides of a controversial issue, and hopefully has done so judiciously. If we could summarize our message in one sentence, it would be that *the ethics of cognitive-enhancing drugs are complex, and cannot be mapped directly onto other drug-related ethical questions such as narcotic abuse or the use of steroids in sports.* There is no substitute for an informed consideration of the relevant facts. The topic is important given the increasing lifestyle use of cognitive-enhancing drugs, and one that—we suspect—will become more pressing in the future as science progresses.

Is it only a matter of time before the nightmare scenario that neuroethicists feared—one filled with academic doping, lifestyle misuse, and 24/7 workdays—becomes reality? Or is the threat being overblown, along with the potential? One thing is certain: executives, academics, and students are seeking a high-impact pill that has minimal side effects, and researchers are doing their best to provide one, because the financial benefit would be tremendous to the pharmaceutical company that develops the ideal 'smart pill' [135]. These medications are being developed to help patients with cognitive impairment, but if benefits are seen in healthy individuals, who or what will stop them from capitalizing on these benefits: conscience; finance; a sense of satisfaction with oneself as is; government regulation?

One abstract concern that is nonetheless a crucial consideration to the parties involved in this debate: should cognitive imperfection be treated as a symptom? A 'quick-fix' pill masks the problem at the heart of poor cognitive performance—perhaps lack of sleep or poor work–life balance—and treats the symptoms just like any other medication. Intellectual strengths have always differed from person to person, and a pill that promises to minimize those differences could be attractive to those who, for example, want to work a little more efficiently or productively. No matter what medications are available, there will almost certainly continue to be a bell curve of human intellect. However, cognitive enhancers may be of great benefit to society as a whole, and particularly the aging population.

Finally, quick-fix solutions risk becoming regarded as the only solution: taking a pill ignores all the other ways that cognition can be enhanced: education, life experience, exercise, healthy diets. Whatever your stance on the ethical questions we have raised here, we believe everyone can agree that it would be a true tragedy if these medications came to replace intellectual development through lifelong learning, or resulted in an over-reliance on a pill to fix one's work–life balance.

We do not feel that scientific inquiry into this subject should cease. On the contrary, the amount of energy and attention paid to the subject will—we hope—increase. At this juncture, it is even more important for society to be engaged in discussions about the pros and cons of these medications, as well as the realities of the lifestyle misuse that already exists. These medications have the potential to change society in dramatic and unexpected ways. Now is the time to have informed discussion and debate of the ethics of these 'smart drugs' and the role they should play in our future society.

CONCLUDING THOUGHTS

I am turned into a sort of machine for observing facts and grinding out conclusions.   Charles Darwin, scientist

When this book was first conceived, we hoped it would bring certain ethical issues regarding smart drugs into the public domain. However, as we set about writing it, we realized that current issues regarding these smart drugs could not be evaluated without a framework of knowledge about the brain and cognitive treatments, and as a result we have tried to provide the necessary framework for interpreting the most current data, and critiquing them with a cautious eye.

The first chapter introduced the literature on normal decision making. Many of the concepts introduced seem intuitive now but were the cause of great debate and discussion when initially proposed. By understanding some of the basic concepts about normal decision making, we were in a better position to later review how decision making is abnormal in certain patient populations.

Chapter 2 discussed scientific ways in which we might be able to explore topics in the neurosciences, including decision making. Tools such as CT, MRI, fMRI, and PET have made it possible for researchers to peer into the mind and begin to elucidate the mysterious functions of the brain. For instance, we and our colleagues have developed two computer tasks that can independently evaluate 'hot' and 'cold' decision making. Moreover, we have discovered that emotional decisions and non-emotional decisions seem to be mediated by different parts of the brain. Even more telling, perhaps, is that people who have had injury to these particular parts of the brain are quite bad at performing tasks of hot and cold decision making.

Next, we reviewed the affective spectrum, and the influence of extreme emotions on decision making. We looked at the physiological changes that might occur when a person feels an emotion such as anger. Using this example, we discussed the ways in which the same physio-logic reactions can lead to different behavioural outcomes in different people, or in the same person in different situations. Emotions are nec-essary for normal cognitive function, but they can also be destructive. A balance of emotional and non-emotional is key, and being either too rational or too emotional can impede our effective functioning.

Using happiness and sadness as an example, we introduced the idea that emotions lie on a continuum. Whilst most individuals are within the part of the continuum that is considered normal, some people live on the polar ends of the continuum. It is unclear why some people experience extreme emotions, but many well-respected people throughout history have done so. Nearer the end of Chapter 3, we discussed a smaller population of individuals who have reduced affective response to circumstances surrounding their daily lives. These individuals suffer from disorders such as Asperger's syndrome. While these children often suffer in their interpersonal interactions, they do so differently from those with extreme emotions.

Taken together, the disorders presented in Chapter 3—especially mania and depression—are ones that we explored when investigat-ing the ways in which extreme emotions can negatively impact deci-sion making. Individuals with mania and depression seem to have disrupted activity in the orbitofrontal areas of their brains (the same areas seemingly used to make emotionally charged decisions) and dorsolateral areas (used for non-emotional decision making). It is not surprising, then, that individuals with mania and depression might make riskier decisions than the normal populations. Some data also suggest that depressed and manic patients may have difficulty with non-emotional decision making: they take longer to make decisions, and as decisions become more difficult, may respond more impulsively. In addition, individuals with damage to their orbitofrontal brain regions also show abnormal decision making during hot tasks, while cold decision making remains intact. Other neurological patients have similar damage to orbitofrontal regions, and similar deficits in emotional decision making.

Chapter 3 ended with the question of whether treatments exist that could attenuate the risky and impulsive decisions that individuals make, and Chapter 4 answered this question with a qualified yes. Cognitive-enhancing medications do exist, though they are not ideal for enhancing all aspects of function, nor for completely restoring patients with neuropsychiatric disorders or brain injury to their original level of functioning. Still, the benefits of these cognitive-enhancing drugs can be of considerable clinical importance. Impulsive behaviour is improved, timeliness of decisions is better, patients can focus longer, among other benefits. Future novel drugs may provide even more effective cognitive enhancement for patients with cognitive impairments. However, research studies have demonstrated that healthy individuals also seem to get some cognitive benefit from taking these medications.

Chapter 5 focused on the concerns surrounding these medications, including the ready availability of non-prescription drugs on the Internet; questions of who should regulate pharmaceutical interventions; discussions of who the recipients of cognitive-enhancing interventions should be; the role of society, the government, researchers, and doctors in shaping the future direction of our cultures.

There is currently a division in public opinion about cognitive-enhancing drugs, at least among the small portion of the population that is engaged with the question at all. Some people imagine that a brain-boosting medication will only provide a negative influence, while others see it as an acceptable—indeed, commendable—means by which to enhance the abilities given to us by nature. The use of drugs to enhance alertness and attention in healthy people is not itself new. Common substances like caffeine and nicotine have some enhancing effects, and are popular at least partly for that reason. However, the increasing lifestyle use of these drugs and the public debate about their use are relatively new. The use of cognitive enhancers is already widespread and surprisingly prevalent [160]. The contentious aspects of this issue will not resolve themselves, and require a well-informed and engaged public to participate in and shape the debate.

ENDNOTES

PREFACE

1. A similar festival—sponsored by the Massachusetts Institute of Technology—exists in Cambridge, Massachusetts and occurs annually in spring.

2. 10 Shattuck Street, Boston, MA 02115. Open Monday to Friday, 9:00–17:00.

3. Phineas Gage was a railway foreman for Rutland and Burlington Rail. One of his responsibilities was to fill drill holes with gunpowder and add a fuse, and then pack in sand with the aid of a tamping iron—a 3 foot 7 inch rod that weighed 13.5 pounds and tapered to a point at one end. On 13 September 1848, Gage neglected to add sand before attempting to tamp down, leaving the gunpowder exposed. The tamping iron struck against the side of the drill hole and sparked, which then ignited the gunpowder and shot the tamping iron into Gage's left cheek under his eye socket and out through the top of his head; it landed approximately 25 yards behind him.

4. Currently, the extent of brain injury is debated, but experts agree the frontal brain was involved.

5. How *drastically* his personality did change is open to conjecture, however. We know very little of Gage's personality before the accident, and what is known about Mr Gage's life after his accident comes largely from a collection of fact, fancy, and fabrication over the years as writers add to the original reports by Dr Harlow. Harlow published two articles on the topic: Passage of an iron rod through the head (1848) *Boston Medical and Surgical Journal*, 39: 389–93; and Recovery from the passage of an iron bar through the head (1868) *Publications of the Massachusetts Medical Society*, 2: 327–47. Harlow made it clear in his 1868 report that Gage's contemporaries found him a changed man. Before his accident, Gage had been one of the company's most capable and efficient workers, but afterwards:

> Gage was fitful, irreverent, indulging at times in the grossest profanity (which was not previously his custom), manifesting but little deference for his fellows, impatient of restraint or advice when it conflicts with his desires, at times pertinaciously obstinate, yet

capricious and vacillating, devising many plans of future operations, which are no sooner arranged than they are abandoned in turn for others appearing more feasible. A child in his intellectual capacity and manifestations, he has the animal passions of a strong man. Previous to his injury, although untrained in the schools, he possessed a well-balanced mind, and was looked upon by those who knew him as a shrewd, smart businessman, very energetic and persistent in executing all his plans of operation. In this regard his mind was radically changed, so decidedly that his friends and acquaintances said he was 'no longer Gage'.

For a more inclusive history of Phineas Gage, see the recent work by M. MacMillon (2000) *An Odd Kind of Fame: Stories of Phineas Gage*, Cambridge, MA: MIT Press.

CHAPTER I

1. It should be said that what is an easy decision for one person in one moment may not be such an easy decision for another person, or in another moment. The context of the decision plays an important role. For instance, deciding to take an umbrella with you when you leave the house is a 'no-brainer' when it is pouring with rain outside. However, the decision might become more difficult if the umbrella is especially cumbersome and it's not raining when you intend to leave the house, but the meteorologist predicts rain with 30 per cent certainty at some point throughout the day.
2. *Oxford English Dictionary.*
3. The reader may not have thought of judgements and decisions as being so complicated since we seem to make them so easily and sometimes without realizing it. However, researchers have investigated different stages of decision and judgement making, which is why we review them here.
4. This feedback is certainly multifaceted, but clearly influenced by the outcome; if a good outcome was achieved, then people usually feel that the judgement or decision was a good one, and the opposite is also true. More information on good decisions and bad decisions can be found in S. L. Schneider and J. Shanteau (eds.), *Emerging perspectives on judgment and decision research* (2003), New York: Cambridge University Press, especially pages 13–63.
5. It has been suggested that many of us make decisions in this way without even realizing it! Also, a group of researchers has confirmed what many others intuitively expected: judgements and decisions become more difficult if attributes conflict (e.g. good quality but expensive cost, or cheap cost but poor quality). See C. P. Haugtvedt, K. Machleit, and R. Talch (eds.), *Online Consumer psychology: Understanding and influencing behavior in the virtual world* (Mahway, NJ: Lawrence Erlbaum, 2005), Mahwah, New Jersey: Lawrence Erlbaum Associates, Inc.

6. In addition, medical students are particularly susceptible to the phenomenon of 'zebra searching', which means that they overestimate the frequency of rare diseases (zebras) and underestimate the frequency of common diseases (horses). This can result in students sometimes believing a rare disorder to be more likely than a common one given a particular set of symptoms. The reader will know, though, that if one hears hoof beats, it's more likely to be from a horse than a zebra. When they are doctors in training, students do not have the clinical wherewithal to have met a large enough patient population to have formed an accurate sense of disease prevalence—their conclusions are based on skewed samples. With experience, this tendency decreases (much to the relief of patients, to be sure!). This tendency to overestimate infrequent events and underestimate frequent events is seen outside the medical profession as well, most notably when asking people about the frequencies of lethal events. The media most likely play a role in sensationalizing rare deaths, causing people to overestimate their frequencies. See Lichtenstein, S., P. Slovic, B. Fischhoff, M. Layman, and B. Coombs (1978) Judged frequency of lethal events, *Journal of Experimental Psychology: Human Learning and Memory*, 4: 551–78. People also tend to recall information that is consistent with the beliefs that they hold, and neglect arguments to the contrary. See Koriat, K., S. Lichtenstein, and B. Fischhoff (1980) Reasons for confidence, *Journal of Experimental Psychology: Human Learning and Memory*, 6: 107–18.

7. As such, different theories of patient treatment have been proposed, from making everything mechanistic and taking the clinical judgement out of all diagnoses, to relying solely on clinical expert judgement. More recently, it has been suggested that clinicians have an important role in deciding which pieces of information are valuable to the overall judgement, and that their role is in this stage of the diagnostic process, whereas the statistical models for combining information should use the information given to them by the clinicians in order to arrive at a more consistently accurate diagnosis. For more information about the clinician's role as the provider of information, the reader can see Dana, J. and R. Thomas (2006) In defense of clinical judgment…and mechanical prediction, *Journal of Behavioral Decision Making*, 19: 413–28; or Einhorn, H. J. (1972) Expert measurement and mechanical combination, *Organizational Behavior and Human Performance*, 7: 86–106.

8. As the authors of the study point out, this promotes interesting speculation about the influence of signs—such as, "Employees must wash hands before returning to work"—or multiple hand-sanitizer stations around a hospital on social attitudes in daily life.

9. Compared averages at http://www.climatetemp.info. In Naples, it is 'wet' 93 days per year but these wet days amount to 919 mm total precipitation. On the other hand, London is 'wet' 164 days per year, but these wet days amount to 594 mm of precipitation.

10. This was further clarified by the psychologists Bar-Hillel and Neter when they studied subordinate and superordinate categorization. See Bar-Hillel, M. and E. Neter (1993) How alike is it versus how likely is it: A disjunction fallacy in probability judgments, *Journal of Personality and Social Psychology*, 65: 1119–31.

11. His book *Words That Work: It's Not What You Say, It's What People Hear* published in 2007 was a *New York Times* bestseller.

12. Original emphasis.

13. See Chapter 2 for a discussion of fMRI.

14. See especially Chapter 8 of the referenced material.

15. This particular quote can be found on page 155 of the referenced work, but the reader is encouraged to read the entirety of Zajonc's argument. Original italics.

16. In the US legal system, a 'crime of passion' is one describing an intensely emotional state of mind induced by some provoking stimulus that could cause a reasonable person to act on impulse or without reflection. This is often considered a mitigating factor in prosecution or sentencing.

CHAPTER 2

1. The Aztecs attempted to localize anger to the liver!

2. This is different from saying that others before this time had ignored the brain. In 1649, René Descartes, for instance, philosophized that anger was the result of spirits agitating the pineal gland.

3. Gall defined twenty-seven such areas, with faculties such as the memory for words, a sense of language, a sense of sound, an instinct for reproduction. Each of these areas was correlated with a bump in the skull, and it was therefore assumed that the degree of mental faculty of a given area could be inferred from studying the enlargements and indentations on an individual's head.

4. Lloyd George prided himself on his knowledge of phrenology and ability to judge a man's character. It has been written that Lloyd George "decided that [Neville Chamberlain's] forehead was too narrow or his skull the wrong shape, and that he had not found a man of the right caliber". See: D. Dilks, (1984) *Neville Chamberlain* Cambridge: Cambridge University Press, p. 195.

5. In November 1891, W. T. Stead wrote of his experience with phrenology in his monthly journal *Review of Reviews*, Volume IV; he and a colleague entered into a competition to see who had the best head/character as determined by a phrenologist.

6. For example, the roughly 100-day Rwandan genocide in 1994 that resulted in the deaths of hundreds of thousands of Tutsi peoples is, in part, thought to have been influenced by early phrenological 'evidence' for racial superiority of one people over another. This 'scientific racism' can be seen in other ethnic purges as well.

7. For instance, in the animated TV series *The Simpsons*, Mr Burns is seen to briefly indulge in phrenology in season 7, episode 8:

BURNS: Who could forget such a monstrous visage? She has the sloping brow and cranial bumpage of the career criminal.

SMITHERS: Uh, Sir? Phrenology was dismissed as quackery 160 years ago.

8. Brodmann's areas are a modern offspring of phrenological thinking, and the brain is divided into approximately fifty such areas based on cytoarchitecture. It is now understood that these areas communicate with each other, and more than one area can be involved in the same function (e.g. execution of a movement).

9. The famous tale of Little Albert fits into a tapestry of early Behavioural experiments that focused on objective responses to stimuli. Little Albert was a child born to a nurse at the Harriet Lane Home for Invalid Children *c*.1920. When Albert was nine months old, researchers presented him with many different objects and animals, including a white rat. It was evident that Albert was quite curious about the white rat, and not at all fearful. Researchers theorized that it was possible to train Albert so that he would become afraid of the rat with which he was previously entranced. Over a series of days, whenever the rat was present, the researchers made an unpleasant loud noise behind Albert's head by using a metal bar to strike a post. This unpleasant noise induced reactions that ranged from surprise to fear and crying. After a few days, the presence of the white rat alone was enough to throw Albert into hysterics. In behavioural terminology, Albert had been *conditioned* to associate unpleasant emotions with the rat.

10. The authors are not suggesting that Behaviourism was a bad thing for science. In fact, it contributed greatly to the backdrop of what has grown into the modern cognitive neurosciences, as well as to psychological treatments for psychiatric disorders (e.g. cognitive behavioural therapy). Fundamentally, however, Behaviourism is not sufficient to understand the human mind and brain functioning, precisely because it ignores an inner mental experience. In other words, we are not automatons solely responding rigidly to particular stimuli. It was Noam Chomsky's critique of Behaviourism in the late 1950s that contributed to the foundation of the cognitive field when he wrote: "[T]he insights that have been achieved in the laboratories of the [Behaviourist], though quite genuine, can be applied to complex human behavior only in the most gross and superficial way," and discussion of language "in these terms alone omit[s] from consideration factors of fundamental importance that are, no doubt, amenable to scientific study, although their specific character cannot at present be precisely formulated". See Chomsky, N. A. (1959) A review of Skinner's verbal behavior, *Language*. 35(1): 26–58.

11. It was Ulric Neisser who defined the phrase 'cognitive psychology' in 1967, although he was not the first to use the terminology. Thomas Verner Moore published a book with the title *Cognitive Psychology* in 1939.

12. The adult brain weighs upwards of 1.3 kilograms (2.9 pounds), and contains billions of *neurons* (see Figure 4). Collections of neurons are *nerves*, and collections of nerves form *pathways*. Roughly three-quarters of the human brain is 'neocortex', otherwise known as the 'new cortex', which lesser animals have not developed to the same extent, and which is not required to survive. Now is not the time nor the place for philosophical banter, but pure survival is assumed to be very different from the existence that we experience. The neocortex is thought to be implicated largely in human consciousness and language, among other things.

13. Researchers were first able to study the different functions of the right and left hemispheres of the brain by observing epilepsy (i.e. seizure) patients who had surgery to sever the band of axons connecting the right and left hemispheres of their brains in a final attempt to control their seizures. Once this procedure is done, the patients' right and left hemispheres cannot communicate with each other, and this resulted in some startling phenomena.

    If given a familiar object to hold (but not see) in their left hand, they would usually be unable to name it. This is because the left hand is connected to the right side/hemisphere of the brain, which has only limited language abilities. However, these 'split-brain' patients *were* recognizing the object even if they couldn't name it; they were able to use their left hands to point out the object within a group of other items. This is one example of the functional deficits that can arise because of anatomical disturbances—in this case the patients really are 'of two minds'.

14. Since anaesthesia was unavailable in psychiatric hospitals at this time, patients were usually rendered unconscious using electroconvulsive therapy. Freeman described his procedure in one patient in very technical terms:

    I introduced the [lobotomy knives] under the eyelids 3 cm from the midline, aimed them parallel with the nose and drove them to a depth of 5 cm. I pulled the handles laterally, returned them halfway and drove them 2 cm deeper. Here I touched the handles over the nose, separated them 45 degrees and elevated them 50 degrees, bringing them parallel for photography before removal.

    Freeman always took a picture of the patient with the lobotomy knives in place. See page 97 in Duffy, H. and C. Fleming (2007) *My Lobotomy*, New York: Crown Publishers.

15. Valerie's "perpetual marble calm" in Sylvia Plath's *The Bell Jar* is one of many literary depictions of the human impact caused by this surgery.

16. See page 99 of the referenced material for quote.

17. One of Freeman's colleagues protested against the lobotomy, stating, "This is not an operation but a mutilation." Another said, "It gave me a sense of horror…How would you like to step into a psychiatrist's office

and have him take out a sterilized ice pick and shove it into the brain over your eyeball? Would you like the idea? No!" See pages 68 and 233 of *My Lobotomy* by H. Dully and C. Fleming.

18. Many other neurointerventional and neurosurgical procedures have been shown to help patients and continue to be used today. For instance, deep brain stimulation is a technique where electrodes are implanted in specific brain locations. It can offer relief to patients with severe movement disorders, and has even shown promise for severely depressed patients. Gamma-knife radiation is a technique used in patients with brain tumours.

19. Broca's area is located in a part of the brain known as the inferior frontal gyrus. There is debate about what other areas are also involved in speech. Although Paul Pierre Broca first noted the deficit in two patients, and post-mortem studies identified lesions in the left lateral frontal lobe, it has since been noted that individuals who have more chronic damage to the area can have preserved speech. See, for instance, Plaza, P. Gatignol, M. Leroy, and H. Duffau (2009) Speaking without Broca's area after tumor resection, *Neurocase*, 9 (2009): 1–17.

20. Wernicke's area is traditionally felt to be located in the superior frontal gyrus of the temporal lobe in the dominant—usually left—hemisphere.

21. If the reader has noticed that the price of helium-filled party balloons has increased and has wondered why this is so, it is in part due to the large demand for liquid helium to cool MRI magnets.

22. The patient listens to the ho–hum–click–click–click of the machine as it works, and some people have even been known to fall asleep.

23. Don't despair! We'll explain. As the radioisotope decays, it emits a positron— a positively charged subatomic particle with a mass identical to an electron. Nearly instantaneously, the positron collides with an electron—its *antimatter*—and the two particles are annihilated, producing a pair of gamma ray photons that then travel in opposite directions. This pair of photons is detected by the scanner around the patient, and it identifies a line, somewhere along which the radioactive decay must have occurred. After thousands upon thousands of collisions are detected, a map of radioactivity is created using intense statistical principles that we won't attempt to describe here.

24. Even neurotransmitters can be radioactively labelled, so that when these molecules bind to their receptors and undergo a radioactive decay, it is possible to see where in the brain certain neurotransmitters act and are concentrated.

25. The relationship between neural activity and blood flow is still being investigated. There is some question about whether blood flow is related more to local field potentials—which reflect a summation of neural activity—than the action potentials of individual neurons that occur when neurons are firing and communicating with neighbours (see Logothetis,

N.K. et al. (2001) Neurophysiological investigation of the basis of the fMRI signal, *Nature*, 412: 150–7). There is also some question about the causal relationship between blood flow and metabolic activity, with some researchers suggesting that blood flow is driven by the presence of neuro-transmitters (see Hyder et al. (2001) Quantitative functional imaging of the brain: towards mapping neuronal activity by BOLD fMRI, *NMR in Bio-medicine*, 14(7–8): 413–31).

26. Changing the strength of the magnet can affect the number and size of signals seen, and also the proportion of small vessels included in the BOLD signal. A 1.5, 2, or 3 Tesla magnet is used.

27. CANTAB was co-invented by Trevor Robbins and Barbara Sahakian, professors at the University of Cambridge. See www.cantab.com and also www.camcog.com.

28. Cognitive studies of risky decision making use two different paradigms. In the first type, the participant understands the outcomes that can result from the decision. In the second type, a decision must be made, but the outcomes are ambiguous. In real-life decisions, these distinctions are less clear.

29. In its classic existence, the Tower of Hanoi has three pegs with a certain number of discs placed in a conical shape—big discs on the bottom and small discs on the top—on one of the three pegs. The goal is to move the entire stack of discs to another peg in the same conical orientation. However, only one disc can be moved at a time, and no disc may be placed on top of a smaller disc. The game was developed in 1883 by French mathematician Édouard Lucas, and was modelled after a legend involving pegs and sixty-four discs found in an Indian temple. According to the legend, when the last disc is moved, the world will end.

30. This computerized version of the Tower of Hanoi task was developed for the CANTAB battery of neuropsychological testing. There now exists the One Touch Stockings of Cambridge for use in neuroimaging studies.

31. Rapid advances in technology have certainly raised some concerns about ramifications of discoveries made using these technologies, and neuroethicists are dealing with questions such as, *Who is the owner of thoughts in a person's consciousness if those thoughts are dangerous—the thinker, or the public?* While nothing can be currently said of a single individual's thoughts, intentions, or mind at this point in scientific discovery, some neuroscientists feel that it is only a matter of time before it becomes possible.

CHAPTER 3

1. Some individuals may also refer to the limbic system as the Papez circuit, though technically this is not correct. The Papez circuit was first described

in 1937 by Dr Papez, and illustrates one of the major pathways within the limbic system. The Papez circuit is likely important in the formation of memories, especially emotionally charged memories.

2. By contrast, as we discussed, cold decision making refers to decisions made in a cool and collected state when emotions are not involved, for example determining the quickest route between point A and point B. This is the rational being, not led astray by emotions. Of course, rational decisions can still be *wrong*.

3. Never mind the fact that IBM's new computer could search up to forty levels of possible moves, with one level corresponding roughly to 80 Elo points, and forty levels corresponding to 3,200 Elo points compared with Kasparov's peak rating of 2,851 Elo points (in chess terms, that is a huge relative skill)!

4. Malcolm Gladwell's book *Blink* (2005) is very good on this subject.

5. Darwin did, however, suggest the relationship and graduated intensity between facial expressions of surprise, astonishment, fear, and ultimately terror.

6. http://www.cdc.gov/Features/dsDepression/ (last accessed 15 Dec 2012).

7. The 'highs' referred to here are manic episodes, which are discussed later in this chapter. If an individual has a manic episode at any point, that individual is said to have bipolar disorder, by definition.

8. These symptoms may be stressful to individuals experiencing them, and recent evidence has shown that prolonged stress can negatively impact the health of the heart. See Grawe, H., M. Katoh, and H. P. Kühl (2006) Stress cardiomyopathy mimicking acute coronary syndrome: case presentation and review of the literature, *Clinical Research in Cardiology*. 95(3): 179–85. In a similar vein, there is an increased death rate in widowers that is suspected to be secondary to cardiovascular disease (in the form of a heart attack) within six months of their spouses' passing. See Hart, C. L. et al. (2007) Effect of conjugal bereavement on mortality of the bereaved spouse in participants of the Renfrew/Paisley Study, *Journal of Epidemiology and Community Health*. 61(5): 455–60. The cardiac principles behind such 'heartbreak' can be more generally applied to the prolonged stress of psychiatric conditions. Thus, it comes as no huge surprise that the risk of cardiovascular disease in depressed individuals is higher than in the general population. See Glassman, A. H. (2007) Depression and cardiovascular comorbidity, *Dialogues in Clinical Neuroscience*, 9(1):9–17.

9. Psychiatric conditions are diagnosed according to a set of criteria laid down by the American Psychiatric Association (APA) which publishes the *Diagnostic and Statistical Manual of Mental Disorders*, currently in its 4th (revised) edition (DSM-IV-TR). The DSM-V is scheduled for release in 2013.

10. In a letter written to Churchill's wife, Clementine, in 1911 after hearing that a friend had been cured of depression by a physician.

11. See page 354 of referenced material for quote.

12. Written in a letter on 23 January 1841 from Abraham Lincoln to John T. Stuart, his first law partner. For a more in-depth appraisal of Lincoln's melancholy

periods, the reader should consider perusing *Lincoln's Melancholy: How Depression Challenged a President and Fueled His Greatness* (2006) by Joshua Wolf Shenk.

13. It is said that originally Joseph Heller intended to refer to a situation in which a character's attempts to avoid a fate simultaneously ensure it as a 'Catch-18' rather than a 'Catch-22', but he had to change the phrase due to copyright issues. This must rank as one of the great instances of literary serendipity, because it's doubtful that the phrase would have entered the cultural lexicon without its endearing alliterative consonance. See. Nagel, (1996) The early composition history of Catch 22, in *Biographies of Books: The Compositional Histories of Notable American Writings*, ed. Barbour and Quirk Columbia, MO: University of Missouri Press.

14. Pease note that Beck's cognitive model of depression is only one model. However, treatment for depression based on this model has been reported to be effective.

15. Confusingly, an individual who has had one episode of mania without depression is also said to have bipolar disorder, since many people with at least one episode of mania go on to experience at least one episode of clinical depression.

16. Lady Caroline Lamb was Lord Byron's cousin by marriage and partner in a lurid and well-publicized love affair in 1812.

17. If interested, the reader should read *An Unquiet Mind, Touched with Fire: Manic Depressive Illness and the Artistic Temperament*, or *Night Falls Fast: Understanding Suicide*, all written by the illustrious Dr Kay Redfield Jamison.

18. Panic attacks, phobias, and panic disorder are often difficult to distinguish from one another, but all are separate disorders with distinct DMS-IV-TR criteria. Hopefully a scenario may serve to elucidate the difference. A lady or gentleman is in a situation that triggers intense arousal (the panic attack). Over days/months/years, said individual may have recurring panic attacks and begin to fear the sensation of physiological arousal to the point that they begin to avoid things that they think may be triggering the panic attacks (panic disorder). Sometimes these symptoms can coincide with an irrational and intense fear of being in a situation from which they cannot escape (agoraphobia).

19. Fear of speaking in public is more common even that fear of death. Thus, as the Jerry Seinfeld joke goes: "According to most studies, people's number one fear is public speaking. Number two is death. Now this means, to the average person, if you have to go to a funeral, you're better off in the casket than doing the eulogy."

20. An alternative therapy is flooding/exposure, which is a faster and more traumatic way of treating phobias than desensitization. In flooding, a psychologist or psychiatrist places the patient in a situation where they are exposed to their phobia at its worst (for instance, if one is afraid of bridges, the therapist

might have the patient walk over a bridge). The exposure can be real, virtual reality, or imagined. The psychiatrist or psychologist then uses relaxation techniques to help the patient calm him- or herself. Once the adrenaline finishes coursing through the patient's system (theoretically time-limited), the patient will calm down and realize there is nothing to fear.

21. If interested, consider reading an essay entitled "Mirror neurons and imitation learning as the driving force behind 'the great leap forward' in human evolution" by Dr Ramachandran in *Edge* web publications (last accessed December 2012): http://www.edge.org/3rd_culture/ramachandran/ ramachandran_p1.html.

22. For an interesting blog about succeeding with Asperger's syndrome, see Penelope Trunk's blog (last accessed September 2012): http://blog.penelopetrunk.com/asperger-syndrome/.

23. Although the prevalence is increasing—mostly due to the fact that more people are living longer—there are some data to suggest that the dementia incidence (the number of new cases diagnosed each year) decreased between 1990 and 2005. See Schrijvers, E.M.C. et al. (2012) Is dementia incidence declining?: Trends in dementia incidence since 1990 in the Rotterdam Study, *Neurology*, 78(19): 1456–63.

24. These memory systems are more accurately located within the hippocampal formation, which is located in the medial aspect of the temporal lobes bilaterally. From an anatomical perspective, the hippocampus has been likened to a sea horse, or *hippocampus* in Latin.

25. For the sake of comparison, the prevalence of tuberculosis in the United Kingdom is approximately 14 per 100,000 people—it is even higher in London at 40 per 100,000. See Burki, T. (2010) Tackling tuberculosis in London's homeless population, *Lancet*, 376(9758): 2055–6.

26. For anyone interested in neurological case histories of patients with frontotemporal dementia, *The Banana Lady and Other Stories of Curious Behavior and Speech* by Andrew Kurtesz provides interesting and factual stories that represent typical behaviours seen in these patients.

27. For example, the neurotransmitter serotonin has been implicated in the presence of depressive symptoms. This finding led to the development of common antidepressant medications, such as Prozac.

28. Bipolar patients do not show the same emotional bias. See Rubinsztein, J.S. et al. (2006) Impaired cognition and decision-making in bipolar depression but no 'affective bias' evident, *Psychological Medicine*, 36(5): 629–39.

29. This area of the brain has been the site of deep brain stimulation in patients with treatment-resistant depression. See Mayberg et al. (2005) Deep brain stimulation for treatment-resistant depression, *Neuron*, 45(5): 651–60. Deep brain stimulation is a neurosurgical procedure that results in an electrode being implanted deep within the brain. When the electrode is turned on, it

alters brain activity, and is used to treat pharmacologically resistant disorders such as Parkinson's disease, hemiballismus, and, more recently, depression.

30. All of the studies we discuss here compare brain activity in the patient (subject) and a healthy volunteer who has no known psychiatric illness (control).

31. The authors have met people who say that during their manic episodes they *do* think that they can fly, and have known others who have jumped from building tops and bridges. Magical thinking such as this is more often seen in patients who have concurrent psychotic symptoms. Psychosis (e.g. the presence of psychotic symptoms, magical thinking, ideas of grandeur) can accompany mania, but does not need to be present for a person to be diagnosed as having a manic episode. The presence of psychotic symptoms has itself been shown to impair the ability to assess risk. See Hutton, S. B. et al. (2002) Decision-making deficits in patients with first-episode and chronic schizophrenia, *Schizophrenia Research*, 55(3): 249–57. People experiencing episodes of mania without psychotic symptoms, however, may also participate in behaviours that lead to self-harm or endangerment.

32. Individuals with this brain injury also do not develop a physiologic skin response prior to risky decisions (e.g. sweaty palms), which is in direct opposition to the skin response seen in healthy volunteers. See Bechara, A. et al. (1996) Failure to respond autonomically to anticipated future outcomes following damage to prefrontal cortex, *Cerebral Cortex*, 6(2): 215–25. One interpretation is that their 'fight or flight' nervous system is off kilter. This is important because they are not even having a physiological reaction to making risky decisions, which may influence their ability to learn from their risky decisions and avoid re-making decisions that had negative consequences in the past.

CHAPTER 4

1. This chapter only reviews some of the various treatments that are available. The ethics of patient care ensure that patient autonomy is always respected, so a patient with capacity to do so can refuse treatment.

2. A procedure invented at Johns Hopkins University in 1937.

3. When the subarachnoid haemorrhage is thought to be the result of an unstable anterior communicating artery (ACoA) aneurysm, this collection of symptoms can be referred to as 'ACoA syndrome'.

4. Which are different in a very important way from illicit stimulants such as cocaine ('coke', 'crack') or (meth)amphetamines ('crystal', 'speed', 'uppers').

5. meth-il-fen'-i-date.

6. Another stimulant used to treat ADHD is Adderall, which contains a mixture of amphetamines, including dextroamphetamine.

7. From the DEA Congressional Testimony on 16 May 2000. Statement by Terrance Woodworth, Deputy Director Office of Diversion Control, Drug Enforcement Administration.

8. Selective serotonin reuptake inhibitors are believed to have a beneficial effect on cognitive function via their ability to improve mood in depressed individuals—indeed, that is their main function—but there have not been extensive studies about the particular cognitive changes seen.

9. This downside of methylphenidate has to do with the way the medication acts. It achieves its effects in part due to its action on dopamine neurotransmitter receptors, and these receptors are also implicated in the mechanism of how your brain interprets rewards and euphoria. See Volkow, N. D. and Swanson, J. M. (2003) Variables that affect the clinical use and abuse of methylphenidate in the treatment of ADHA, *American Journal of Psychiatry*, 160(11): 1909–18.

10. moe-daf'-i-nil; modafinil, also known as Provigil, has a decreased number of serious side effects when compared with methylphenidate, but nor has it been in use long enough for the long-term effects on healthy (i.e. non-narcoleptic) individuals to be known. Headache, dizziness, and anxiety are the most often reported side effects.

11. Modafinil—similar to other addictive medications like methylphenidate—acts on dopamine and norepinephrine neurotransmitter receptors. See Minzenberg et al. (2008) Modafinil shifts human locus coeruleus to low-tonic, high-phasic activity during functional MRI, *Science*, 322(5908): 1700–2; and also Volkow et al. (2009) Effects of modafinil on dopamine and dopamine transporters in the male human brain: clinical implications, *JAMA*, 301(11): 1148–54. Modafinil also has effects on histamine and glutamate. See Scoriels et al. (2013) Modafinil effects on cognition and emotion in schizophrenia and its neurochemical modulation in the brain, *Neuropharmacology*, 64:168–84.

12. Dr James Maas is a recently retired sleep specialist who taught at Cornell University in Ithaca, NY. Ironically, his popular morning class was attended by tens of thousands of sleep-deprived students over the many years of his career. More than 65,000 students have taken this class since its inception.

13. It used to be thought that dreams only occurred during REM sleep, but this turns out not to be the case. For more interesting dream facts, it would be worth exploring 'How dreams work' at http://science.howstuffworks.com/ (last accessed September 2012)

14. It is well known that various countries' military branches have used Dexedrine (Dextroamphetamine) to successfully increase wakefulness in military personnel. See Caldwell, J. A., Caldwell, J. L. et al. (1995) Sustaining helicopter pilot performance with Dexedrine during periods of sleep deprivation, *Aviation, Space, and Environmental Medicine*, 66(10): 930–7; and Caldwell, J. A. and J. L. Caldwell (1997) An in-flight investigation of the efficacy of Dextroamphetamine for sustaining helicopter

pilot performance, *Aviation, Space, and Environmental Medicine*, 68(12): 1073–80. Dexedrine is more powerful than amphetamine, but slightly less potent than methamphetamine. However, it has a very high potential for abuse, and therefore other less habit-forming alternatives or add-on therapies have recently been investigated by the military. Modafinil is thought to be an appropriate candidate given the similar behavioural and subjective effects between modafinil and dextroamphetamine, and the decreased side-effect profile at effective doses. See Makris, A. P., C. R. Rush, et al. (2004) Wake-promoting agents with different mechanisms of action: comparison of effects of Modafinil and Amphetamine on food intake and cardiovascular activity, *Appetite*, 42(2): 185–95; and Makris, A. P., C. R. Rush, et al. (2007) Behavioral and subjective effects of d-amphetamine and Modafinil in healthy adults, *Experimental and Clinical Psychopharmacology*, 15(2): 123–33.

CHAPTER 5

1. This chapter contains material revised from commentaries that appeared in *Nature*. See Sahakian, B. and S. Morein-Zamir (2007) Professor's Little helper, *Nature*, 450(20): 1157–9. Our discussion in this chapter is also influenced by another *Nature* publication; see Greely, H., B. Sahakian, J. Harris, R. C. Kessler, M. Gazzaniga, P. Campbell, and M. J. Farah (2008) Towards responsible use of cognitive-enhancing drugs by the healthy, *Nature*, 456(7223): 702–5.

2. A separate discussion is currently occurring with regard to non-pharmacologic forms of cognitive enhancement. Recently, the concept of transcranial direct current stimulation has received public attention. Transcranial direct current stimulation uses electrodes that are placed on the outside of the skull to pass small amounts of electricity through to the brain for a period of minutes. If this is done while someone is—for example—reading, participating in math lessons, or even sharpshooting, learning seems to be improved. The theory behind these improvements is that the small amount of current makes it easier for the neurons to fire, and that this added brain activity enhances and strengthens connections between brain areas. It is reportedly painless, and most of the research so far has been carried out in healthy adults. The technique would require standard education and training, but reportedly enables people to get more out of the learning 'process'. See Adee, S. (2012) Zap your brain into the zone: fast track to pure focus, *New Scientist*, 6 (2850).

3. The majority of these stimulants are Schedule I—highly illegal and abused compounds—with the exception of methylphenidate (Schedule II) and modafinil (Schedule IV). Scheduled drugs are controlled substances with abuse potential, although alcohol, tobacco, and caffeine are specifically excluded. There is some debate about the appropriate process for deciding

which drugs end up in which schedule (I–V); at present, a drug's schedule class does not always align with its potential for harm.

4. In the recent movie *Limitless* (2011), Edward Morra is down on his luck until he comes across a new type of smart drug, NZT-48. This particular cognitive enhancer (which is fictional, mind you) allows humans to access 100 per cent of their brainpower, as opposed to the normal, lower level of activation (this is also a common myth—there are no 'unused' parts of the brain). The drug works, and works well. Unfortunately, despite his success, Edward begins to show behaviours of drug abuse. He increases his dose of the drug, which causes side effects including lost time, frenetic activity, and heart palpitations. The drug itself seems to give Edward a sort of intelligence superpower that, when discovered by other people, causes him more problems than he would ever have imagined before he comes to his senses and limits his reliance on the drug.

5. For example, there's an app that allows someone first to purchase a plane ticket, check in for the flight, and display a boarding pass, all from a mobile phone. At the risk of dating ourselves: unbelievable.

6. At the doses that produce effective alertness, there are common side effects such as tremor.

7. Even though these patients' test scores improved following the nicotine patches, their overall global functioning did not improve in any statistically relevant manner.

8. *Leviathan*, Ch. 13, para. 9.

9. This phenomenon is also apparent in popular culture, as more entertainment media are incorporating lifestyle use into their plots. For instance, in season 1, episode 3 of the TV series *Lie to Me*, a judge's daughter is portrayed as using methylphenidate to help herself study more effectively in order to get better grades/test scores and be admitted to a better university.

10. Short-term side effects of modafinil include headache, nausea, nervousness, anxiety, and insomnia.

11. The efficacy of bans and warnings is also inversely proportional to their prevalence. For instance, since the passage of a ballot measure called Proposition 65 in 1986, many products (*many* products) sold in California now carry a tag stating "WARNING: This product contains chemicals known to the State of California to cause cancer and birth defects or other reproductive harm." Seeing this warning on everything has not necessarily made Californians more able to avoid potentially hazardous products.

12. It is possible to buy Ritalin (or what the Internet source claims is Ritalin) online for as little as 40 pence (approximately $0.65) a tablet, and one can purchase modafinil (or, again, what claims to be modafinil) tablets online for 50 pence (approximately $0.75) each. We hardly think it should be necessary to say so, but just to be very clear: DO NOT buy such medications from online sources without a prescription.

13. Dr Chatterjee, an educator at the University of Pennsylvania, recalls a time when a similar attitude was expressed against cosmetic surgery for beautification and self-image purposes; now, though, cosmetic surgery is practically a mainstream entity. You can even get botox injections from your dermatologist. See Carey, B. (2008) Brain enhancement is wrong, right? in *The New York Times* (9 March).

ACKNOWLEDGEMENTS

This book has been a true group effort, with many people playing various roles.

Thank you to Dr Andrew Blackwell, Miranda Robbins, Jacqueline Robbins, and Dr Sharon Morein-Zamir for assisting with the slide presentation for the original lectures. The authors are grateful to Dr Samuel Chamberlain for initial discussion on the organization for the book, on which we were able to expound. Thank you to Professor Trevor Robbins for his helpful comments on the final manuscript. Thanks also go to Dr Evan LaBuzetta for reading, commenting upon, and rereading the various iterations of this text.

In addition, Jamie LaBuzetta would like to thank her family, who has always supported her whims and pushed her to follow her dreams. You have been patient and loving—a steadfast base of support, and a beacon of light when she yearned for *home*. To her husband, she would like to say: your endless support and language skills leave me speechless, particularly if you are not helping me to find the 'write' words.

Much of the research included in this book was completed with the aid of a Wellcome Trust grant and within the Medical Research Council and Wellcome Trust Behavioural and Clinical Neurosciences Institute.

The Cambridge Gamble Task and Stockings of Cambridge Task are part of the CANTAB tests, Cambridge Cognition Limited (www.camcog.com). Professor Sahakian is a consultant for Cambridge Cognition Limited. Trevor Robbins and Barbara Sahakian are co-inventors of CANTAB.

REFERENCES

1. Sahakian, B. J. and S. Morein-Zamir, Neuroscientists need neuroethics teaching. *Science*, 2009. **325**(5937): pp. 147.
2. Labuzetta, J. N., R. Burnstein, and J. Pickard, Ethical issues in consenting vulnerable patients for neuroscience research. *Journal of psychopharmacology*, 2011. **25**(2): pp. 205–10.
3. Klayman, J., Cue discovery in probabilistic environments. *Acta Psychologica*, 1988. **56**: pp. 81–92.
4. Connolly, T. and B. K. Thorn, Predecisional information acquisition: effects of task variables on suboptimal search strategies. *Organizational Behavior and Human Decision Processes*, 1987. **39**: pp. 397–416.
5. Hershman, R. L. and J. R. Levine, Deviations from optimal purchase strategies in human decision making. *Organizational Behavior and Human Performance*, 1970. **5**: pp. 313–29.
6. Simon, H. A., Rational choice and the structure of the environment. *Psychol Rev*, 1956. **63**(2): pp. 129–38.
7. Meehl, P., Clinical Versus Statistical Prediction: A Theoretical Analysis and a Review of the Evidence. 1956, Minneapolis: University of Minnesota Press.
8. Promberger, M. and J. Baron, Do patients trust computers? *Journal of Behavioral Decision Making*, 2006. **19**: pp. 455–68.
9. Helzer, E. G. and D. A. Pizarro, Dirty liberals! Reminders of physical cleanliness influence moral and political attitudes. *Psychological Science*, 2011. **22**(4): pp. 517–22.
10. Kahneman, D. and A. Tversky, On the study of statistical intuitions. *Cognition*, 1982. **11**(2): pp. 123–41.
11. McNeil, B. J., et al., On the elicitation of preferences for alternative therapies. *N Engl J Med*, 1982. **306**(21): pp. 1259–62.
12. Frank Luntz Interview (15 December 2003). Last updated: 9 November 2004. Accessed 12 September 2012; available from: http://www.pbs.org/wgbh/pages/frontline/shows/persuaders/interviews/luntz.html.
13. Luntz, F., The New American Lexicon, 2006.
14. Mishra, S., M. Gregson, and M. L. Lalumiere, Framing effects and risk-sensitive decision making. *British Journal of Psychology*, 2012. **103**(1): pp. 83–97.

15. Samuelson, W. and R. Zeckhauser, Status quo bias in decision making. *Journal of Risk and Uncertainty*, 1988. **1**(1): pp. 7–59.
16. Hariri, A. R., et al., Preference for immediate over delayed rewards is associated with magnitude of ventral striatal activity. *J Neurosci*, 2006. **26**(51): pp. 13213–17.
17. McClure, S. M., et al., Separate neural systems value immediate and delayed monetary rewards. *Science*, 2004. **306**(5695): pp. 503–7.
18. Ward, A. and T. Mann, Don't mind if I do: disinhibited eating under cognitive load. *J Pers Soc Psychol*, 2000. **78**(4): pp. 753–63.
19. Wolfe, T., The Right Stuff. 1979, New York: Picador.
20. Damasio, A. R., The somatic marker hypothesis and the possible functions of the prefrontal cortex. *Philos Trans R Soc Lond B Biol Sci*, 1996. **351**(1346): pp. 1413–20.
21. Zajonc, R., Feeling and thinking: preferences need no inferences. *American Psychologist*, 1980. **35**: pp. 151–75.
22. Roiser, J. P., J. S. Rubinsztein, and B. J. Sahakian, Neuropsychology of affective disorders. *Psychiatry*, 2008. **8**(3): pp. 91–6.
23. Ariely, D. and G. Loewenstein, The heat of the moment: the effect of sexual arousal on sexual decision making. *Journal of Behavioral Decision Making*, 2006. **19**: pp. 87–98.
24. Caruso, E. M. and E. Shafir, Now that I think about it, I'm in the mood for laughs: decisions focused on mood. *Journal of Behavioral Decision Making*, 2006. **19**: pp. 155–69.
25. Dully, H. and C. Fleming, My Lobotomy. 2007, New York: Crown Publishers.
26. Lorenzetti, V., et al., Structural brain abnormalities in major depressive disorder: a selective review of recent MRI studies. *Journal of Affective Disorders*, 2009. **117**(1–2): pp. 1–17.
27. Aron, A., et al., Politics and the brain, in *The New York Times*, 14 November 2007.
28. Haynes, J. D. and G. Rees, Decoding mental states from brain activity in humans. *Nature reviews. Neuroscience*, 2006. **7**(7): pp. 523–34.
29. O'Doherty, J. E., et al., Active tactile exploration using a brain-machine-brain interface. *Nature*, 2011. **479**(7372): pp. 228–31.
30. Baker, S. C., et al., Neural systems engaged by planning: a PET study of the Tower of London task. *Neuropsychologia*, 1996. **34**(6): pp. 515–26.
31. Manes, F., et al., Decision-making processes following damage to the prefrontal cortex. *Brain*, 2002. **125**(Pt 3): pp. 624–39.
32. Rogers, R. D., et al., Choosing between small, likely rewards and large, unlikely rewards activates inferior and orbital prefrontal cortex. *J Neurosci*, 1999. **19**(20): pp. 9029–38.
33. Kahneman, D. and A. Tversky, Choices, Values, Frames. 2000, Cambridge, UK: Cambridge University Press.

34. Lawrence, A., et al., The innovative brain. *Nature*, 2008. **456**(7219): pp. 168–9.
35. Kotler, S. Training the brain of an entrepreneur. *Forbes*, 2012. Accessed 6 November 2012; available from: http://www.forbes.com/sites/stevenkotler/2012/05/14/training-the-brain-of-an-entrepreneur/.
36. Parker-Pope, T., Maternal instinct is wired into the brain, in *The New York Times*, 7 March 2008.
37. Blackslee, S., If Your Brain Has a 'Buy Button,' What Pushes It?, in *The New York Times*, 19 October 2004.
38. Sample, I., The brain scan that can read people's intentions: call for ethical debate over possible use of new technology in interrogation, in *The Guardian*, 9 February 2007.
39. Erickson, K., et al., Mood-congruent bias in affective go/no-go performance of unmedicated patients with major depressive disorder. *Am J Psychiatry*, 2005. **162**(11): pp. 2171–3.
40. Styron, W., Darkness Visible: A Memoir of Madness. 1990, New York: Random House.
41. Scott, W., The Journal of Sir Walter Scott, ed. W. E. K. Anderson. 1972, Oxford: Clarendon Press.
42. Landau, E. Experts ponder link between creativity, mood disorders. Last updated: 2 April 2009. Accessed 12 September 2012; available from: http://edition.cnn.com/2008/HEALTH/conditions/10/07/creativity.depression/index.html.
43. Verhaeghen, P., J. Joorman, and R. Khan, Why we sing the blues: the relation between self-reflective rumination, mood, and creativity. *Emotion*, 2005. **5**(2): pp. 226–32.
44. Roiser, J. P., R. Elliott, and B. J. Sahakian, Cognitive mechanisms of treatment in depression. *Neuropsychopharmacology*: official publication of the American College of Neuropsychopharmacology, 2012. **37**(1): pp. 117–36.
45. Davison, G. C., and J. M. Neale, Abnormal Psychology: An Experimental Clinical Approach. 1986, New York: John Wiley & Sons.
46. Kolk, L. C., Modern Clinical Psychiatry (8th edn). 1973, Philadelphia: W.B. Saunders.
47. Gorelick, P., Risk factors for vascular dementia and Alzheimer disease. *Stroke*, 2004. **35**(11 Suppl): pp. 2620–2.
48. Ferri, C. P., et al., Global prevalence of dementia: a Delphi consensus study. *Lancet*, 2005. **366**(9503): pp. 2112–17.
49. Ratnavalli, E., et al., The prevalence of frontotemporal dementia. *Neurology*, 2002. **58**(11): pp. 1615–21.
50. Elliott, R., et al., The neural basis of mood-congruent processing biases in depression. *Arch Gen Psychiatry*, 2002. **59**(7): pp. 597–604.
51. Elliott, R., et al., Abnormal ventral frontal response during performance of an affective go/no go task in patients with mania. *Biol Psychiatry*, 2004. **55**(12): pp. 1163–70.

52. Drevets, W. C., et al., A functional anatomical study of unipolar depression. *J Neurosci*, 1992. **12**(9): pp. 3628–41.
53. Drevets, W. C., J. Savitz, and M. Trimble, The subgenual anterior cingulate cortex in mood disorders. *CNS Spectrums*, 2008. **13**(8): pp. 663–81.
54. Murphy, F. C., et al., Decision-making cognition in mania and depression. *Psychol Med*, 2001. **31**(4): pp. 679–93.
55. Rubinsztein, J. S., et al., Impaired cognition and decision-making in bipolar depression but no 'affective bias' evident. *Psychol Med*, 2006. **36**(5): pp. 629–39.
56. Jollant, F., et al., Impaired decision making in suicide attempters. *Am J Psychiatry*, 2005. **162**(2): pp. 304–10.
57. Kyte, Z. A., I. M. Goodyer, and B. J. Sahakian, Selected executive skills in adolescents with recent first episode major depression. *J Child Psychol Psychiatry*, 2005. **46**(9): pp. 995–1005.
58. Murphy, F. C., et al., Emotional bias and inhibitory control processes in mania and depression. *Psychol Med*, 1999. **29**(6): pp. 1307–21.
59. Elliott, R., et al., Abnormal response to negative feedback in unipolar depression: evidence for a diagnosis specific impairment. *J Neurol Neurosurg Psychiatry*, 1997. **63**(1): pp. 74–82.
60. Murphy, F. C., et al., Neuropsychological impairment in patients with major depressive disorder: the effects of feedback on task performance. *Psychol Med*, 2003. **33**(3): pp. 455–67.
61. Rogers, R. D., et al., Dissociable deficits in the decision-making cognition of chronic amphetamine abusers, opiate abusers, patients with focal damage to prefrontal cortex, and tryptophan-depleted normal volunteers: evidence for monoaminergic mechanisms. *Neuropsychopharmacology*, 1999. **20**(4): pp. 322–39.
62. Clark, L., et al., Differential effects of insular and ventromedial prefrontal cortex lesions on risky decision-making. *Brain*, 2008. **131**(Pt 5): pp. 1311–22.
63. Bechara, A., et al., Insensitivity to future consequences following damage to human prefrontal cortex. *Cognition*, 1994. **50**(1–3): pp. 7–15.
64. Rahman, S., et al., Specific cognitive deficits in mild frontal variant frontotemporal dementia. *Brain*, 1999. **122 (Pt 8)**: pp. 1469–93.
65. Mavaddat, N., et al., Deficits in decision-making in patients with aneurysms of the anterior communicating artery. *Brain*, 2000. **123** (Pt 10): pp. 2109–17.
66. Piotin, M., et al., Intracranial aneurysms: treatment with bare platinum coils—aneurysm packing, complex coils, and angiographic recurrence. *Radiology*, 2007. **243**(2): pp. 500–8.
67. Mavaddat, N., et al., Cognition following subarachnoid hemorrhage from anterior communicating artery aneurysm: relation to timing of surgery. *J Neurosurg*, 1999. **91**(3): pp. 402–7.
68. Frazer, D., et al., Coiling versus clipping for the treatment of aneurysmal subarachnoid hemorrhage: a longitudinal investigation into cognitive outcome. *Neurosurgery*, 2007. **60**(3): pp. 434–41; discussion 441–2.

69. Eagger, S. A., R. Levy, and B. J. Sahakian, Tacrine in Alzheimer's disease. *Lancet*, 1991. **337**(8748): pp. 989–92.

70. Howard, R., et al., Donepezil and memantine for moderate-to-severe Alzheimer's disease. *N Engl J Med*, 2012. **366**(10): pp. 893–903.

71. Yesavage, J. A., et al., Donepezil and flight simulator performance: effects on retention of complex skills. *Neurology*, 2002. **59**(1): pp. 123–5.

72. Gron, G., et al., Cholinergic enhancement of episodic memory in healthy young adults. *Psychopharmacology*, 2005. **182**(1): pp. 170–9.

73. Volkow, N.D., et al., Dopamine transporter occupancies in the human brain induced by therapeutic doses of oral methylphenidate. *Am J Psychiatry*, 1998. **155**(10): pp. 1325–31.

74. Devito, E. E., et al., The effects of methylphenidate on decision making in attention-deficit/hyperactivity disorder. *Biol Psychiatry*, 2008. **64**(7): pp. 636–9.

75. Satel, S. L. and J. C. Nelson, Stimulants in the treatment of depression: a critical overview. *The Journal of Clinical Psychiatry*, 1989. **50**(7): pp. 241–9.

76. Mattes, J. A., Methylphenidate in mild depression: a double-blind controlled trial. *The Journal of Clinical Psychiatry*, 1985. **46**(12): pp. 525–7.

77. Kaplitz, S. E., Withdrawn, apathetic geriatric patients responsive to methylphenidate. *Journal of the American Geriatrics Society*, 1975. **23**(6): pp. 271–6.

78. Hardy, S. E., Methylphenidate for the treatment of depressive symptoms, including fatigue and apathy, in medically ill older adults and terminally ill adults. *The American Journal of Geriatric Pharmacotherapy*, 2009. **7**(1): pp. 34–59.

79. Kerr, C. W., et al., Effects of methylphenidate on fatigue and depression: a randomized, double-blind, placebo-controlled trial. *Journal of Pain and Symptom Management*, 2012. **43**(1): pp. 68–77.

80. El-Mallakh, R. S., An open study of methylphenidate in bipolar depression. *Bipolar Disorders*, 2000. **2**(1): pp. 56–9.

81. Carlson, P. J., M. C. Merlock, and T. Suppes, Adjunctive stimulant use in patients with bipolar disorder: treatment of residual depression and sedation. *Bipolar Disorders*, 2004. **6**(5): pp. 416–20.

82. Lavretsky, H., et al., Combined treatment with methylphenidate and citalopram for accelerated response in the elderly: an open trial. *The Journal of Clinical Psychiatry*, 2003. **64**(12): pp. 1410–14.

83. Leite, W. B., L. F. Malloy-Diniz, and H. Correa, Effects of methylphenidate on cognition and behaviour: ruptured communicant aneurysm of the anterior artery. *Aust N Z J Psychiatry*, 2007. **41**(6): pp. 554–6.

84. Rahman, S., et al., Methylphenidate ('Ritalin') can ameliorate abnormal risk-taking behavior in the frontal variant of frontotemporal dementia. *Neuropsychopharmacology*, 2006. **31**(3): pp. 651–8.

85. Kim, Y. H., et al., Effects of single-dose methylphenidate on cognitive performance in patients with traumatic brain injury: a double-blind placebo-controlled study. *Clin Rehabil*, 2006. **20**(1): pp. 24–30.

86. Whyte, J., et al., Effects of methylphenidate on attention deficits after traumatic brain injury: a multidimensional, randomized, controlled trial. *Am J Phys Med Rehabil*, 2004. **83**(6): pp. 401–20.

87. Lee, H., et al., Comparing effects of methylphenidate, sertraline and placebo on neuropsychiatric sequelae in patients with traumatic brain injury. *Human Psychopharmacology*, 2005. **20**(2): pp. 97–104.

88. Plenger, P. M., et al., Subacute methylphenidate treatment for moderate to moderately severe traumatic brain injury: a preliminary double-blind placebo-controlled study. *Arch Phys Med Rehabil*, 1996. **77**(6): pp. 536–40.

89. Moein, H., H. A. Khalili, and K. Keramatian, Effect of methylphenidate on ICU and hospital length of stay in patients with severe and moderate traumatic brain injury. *Clin Neurol Neurosurg*, 2006. **108**(6): pp. 539–42.

90. Oualtieri, C. T. and R. W. Evans, Stimulant treatment for the neurobehavioural sequelae of traumatic brain injury. *Brain Inj*, 1988. 2(4):p p. 273–90.

91. Meyers, C. A., et al., Methylphenidate therapy improves cognition, mood, and function of brain tumor patients. *J Clin Oncol*, 1998. **16**(7): pp. 2522–7.

92. Galynker, I., et al., Methylphenidate treatment of negative symptoms in patients with dementia. *J Neuropsychiatry Clin Neurosci*, 1997. **9**(2): pp. 231–9.

93. Elliott, R., et al., Effects of methylphenidate on spatial working memory and planning in healthy young adults. *Psychopharmacology (Berl)*, 1997. **131**(2): pp. 196–206.

94. Volkow, N., June 2012. Personal communication.

95. Bray, C. L., et al., Methylphenidate does not improve cognitive function in healthy sleep-deprived young adults. *J Investig Med*, 2004. **52**(3): pp. 192–201.

96. Turner, D. C., et al., Relative lack of cognitive effects of methylphenidate in elderly male volunteers. *Psychopharmacology (Berl)*, 2003. **168**(4): pp. 455–64.

97. Kratochvil, C. J., ADHD pharmacotherapy: rates of stimulant use and cardiovascular risk. *Am J Psychiatry*, 2012. **169**(2): pp. 112–14.

98. McDonagh, M. S., et al., Drug Class Review on Pharmacologic Treatments for ADHD: Final Report 2007: Portland, OR: Oregon Health and Science University.

99. Schelleman, H., et al., Methylphenidate and risk of serious cardiovascular events in adults. *Am J Psychiatry*, 2012. **169**(2): pp. 178–85.

100. O, Billiard, M., et al., Modafinil: a double-blind multicentric study. *Sleep*, 1994. **17**(8 Suppl): pp. S107–12.

101. Amiri, S., et al., Modafinil as a treatment for Attention-Deficit/Hyperactivity Disorder in children and adolescents: a double blind, randomized clinical trial. *Prog Neuropsychopharmacol Biol Psychiatry*, 2008. **32**(1): pp. 145–9.

102. Dackis, C. A., et al., A double-blind, placebo-controlled trial of modafinil for cocaine dependence. *Neuropsychopharmacology*, 2005. **30**(1): pp. 205–11.

103. Morein-Zamir, S., D. C. Turner, and B. J. Sahakian, A review of the effects of modafinil on cognition in schizophrenia. *Schizophr Bull*, 2007. **33**(6): pp. 1298–306.

104. Turner, D. C., et al., Modafinil improves cognition and attentional set shifting in patients with chronic schizophrenia. *Neuropsychopharmacology*, 2004. **29**(7): pp. 1363–73.

105. Nieves, A. V. and A. E. Lang, Treatment of excessive daytime sleepiness in patients with Parkinson's disease with modafinil. *Clin Neuropharmacol*, 2002. **25**(2): pp. 111–14.

106. Rammohan, K. W., et al., Efficacy and safety of modafinil (Provigil) for the treatment of fatigue in multiple sclerosis: a two centre phase 2 study. *J Neurol Neurosurg Psychiatry*, 2002. **72**(2): pp. 179–83.

107. Gebhardt, D. O., Off-label administration of drugs to healthy military personnel: dubious ethics of preventive measures. *J Med Ethics*, 2005. **31**(5): pp. 268.

108. Eliyahu, U., et al., Psychostimulants and military operations. *Mil Med*, 2007. **172**(4): pp. 383–7.

109. Turner, D. C., et al., Modafinil improves cognition and response inhibition in adult attention-deficit/hyperactivity disorder. *Biol Psychiatry*, 2004. **55**(10): pp. 1031–40.

110. Zack, M. and C. X. Poulos, Effects of the atypical stimulant modafinil on a brief gambling episode in pathological gamblers with high vs. low impulsivity. *J Psychopharmacol*, 2008. **23**(6): pp. 660–71.

111. Blackwell, A. D., et al., The effects of modafinil on mood and cognition in Huntington's disease. *Psychopharmacology (Berl)*, 2008. **199**(1): pp. 29–36.

112. Turner, D. C., et al., Cognitive enhancing effects of modafinil in healthy volunteers. *Psychopharmacology (Berl)*, 2003. **165**(3): pp. 260–9.

113. Muller, U., et al., Effects of modafinil on non-verbal cognition, task enjoyment and creative thinking in healthy volunteers. *Neuropharmacology*, 2013. **64**(1): pp. 490–5.

114. Randall, D. C., et al., Does modafinil enhance cognitive performance in young volunteers who are not sleep-deprived? *J Clin Psychopharmacol*, 2005. **25**(2): pp. 175–9.

115. Randall, D. C., et al., The cognitive-enhancing properties of modafinil are limited in non-sleep-deprived middle-aged volunteers. *Pharmacol Biochem Behav*, 2004. **77**(3): pp. 547–55.

116. Randall, D. C., J. M. Shneerson, and S. E. File, Cognitive effects of modafinil in student volunteers may depend on IQ. *Pharmacol Biochem Behav*, 2005. **82**(1): pp. 133–9.

117. Maas, J. B., Power Sleep: The Revolutionary Program that Prepares Your Mind for Peak Performance. 1998, New York: HarperCollins (Quill).

118. Curcio, G., M. Ferrara, and L. De Gennaro, Sleep loss, learning capacity and academic performance. *Sleep Medicine Reviews*, 2006. **10**(5): pp. 323–37.
119. Fido, A. and A. Ghali, Detrimental effects of variable work shifts on quality of sleep, general health and work performance. *Medical Principles and Practice: International Journal of the Kuwait University*, Health Science Centre, 2008. **17**(6): pp. 453–7.
120. Smith, L., S. Folkard, and C. J. Poole, Increased injuries on night shift. *Lancet*, 1994. **344**(8930): pp. 1137–9.
121. Akerstedt, T., Shift work and disturbed sleep/wakefulness. *Occupational Medicine*, 2003. **53**(2): pp. 89–94.
122. Rosekind, M. R., et al., The cost of poor sleep: workplace productivity loss and associated costs. *Journal of Occupational and Environmental Medicine/American College of Occupational and Environmental Medicine*, 2010. **52**(1): pp. 91–8.
123. Belenky, G., L. J. Wu, and M. L. Jackson, Occupational sleep medicine: practice and promise. *Progress in Brain Research*, 2011. **190**: pp. 189–203.
124. Night Working: Return of the Graveyard Shift, in *The Economist*, 15 September 2012.
125. Lockley, S. W., et al., Effects of health care provider work hours and sleep deprivation on safety and performance. *Jt Comm J Qual Patient Saf*, 2007. **33**(11 Suppl): pp. 7–18.
126. Chen, I., et al., A survey of subjective sleepiness and consequences in attending physicians. *Behav Sleep Med*, 2008. **6**(1): pp. 1–15.
127. Gill, M., et al., Cognitive performance following modafinil versus placebo in sleep-deprived emergency physicians: a double-blind randomized crossover study. *Acad Emerg Med*, 2006. **13**(2): pp. 158–65.
128. Sugden, C., et al., Effect of pharmacological enhancement on the cognitive and clinical psychomotor performance of sleep-deprived doctors: a randomized controlled trial. *Annals of Surgery*, 2012. **255**(2): pp. 222–7.
129. Caldwell, J. A., Jr., et al., A double-blind, placebo-controlled investigation of the efficacy of modafinil for sustaining the alertness and performance of aviators: a helicopter simulator study. *Psychopharmacology (Berl)*, 2000. **150**(3): pp. 272–82.
130. Caldwell, J. A., Jr., et al., The efficacy of modafinil for sustaining alertness and simulator flight performance in F-117 pilots during 37 hours of continuous wakefulness, *United States Air Force Research Laboratory*, 2004.
131. Taylor, G. P., Jr. and R. E. Keys, modafinil and Management of Aircrew Fatigue (Memorandum), 2003.
132. Brady, B., MoD's secret pep pill to keep forces awake, in Scotland on Sunday, 27 February 2005: Scotland.
133. Zuvekas, S. H. and B. Vitiello, Stimulant medication use in children: a 12-year perspective. *Am J Psychiatry*, 2012. **169**(2): pp. 160–6.

134. All on the mind, in The Economist, 22 May 2008.

135. Hall, S. S., The quest for a smart pill. *Sci Am*, 2003. **289**(3): pp. 54–7, 60–5.

136. Sahakian, B. J. and S. Morein-Zamir, Professor's little helper. *Nature*, 2007. **450**(20): pp. 1157–59.

137. Comas-Herrera, A., et al., Cognitive impairment in older people: future demand for long-term care services and the associated costs. *Int J Geriatr Psychiatry*, 2007. **22**(10): pp. 1037–45.

138. Bryson, B., I'm a Stranger Here Myself. 1999, New York: Broadway Books.

139. Huck, N. O., et al., The effects of modafinil, caffeine, and dextroamphetamine on judgments of simple versus complex emotional expressions following sleep deprivation. *Int J Neurosci*, 2008. **118**(4): pp. 487–502.

140. Killgore, W. D., et al., Effects of dextroamphetamine, caffeine and modafinil on psychomotor vigilance test performance after 44 h of continuous wakefulness. *J Sleep Res*, 2008. **17**(3): 309–21.

141. Dagan, Y. and J. T. Doljansky, Cognitive performance during sustained wakefulness: a low dose of caffeine is equally effective as modafinil in alleviating the nocturnal decline. *Chronobiol Int*, 2006. **23**(5): pp. 973–83.

142. Wesensten, N. J., W. D. Killgore, and T. J. Balkin, Performance and alertness effects of caffeine, dextroamphetamine, and modafinil during sleep deprivation. *J Sleep Res*, 2005. **14**(3): pp. 255–66.

143. Wesensten, N. J., et al., Maintaining alertness and performance during sleep deprivation: modafinil versus caffeine. *Psychopharmacology (Berl)*, 2002. **159**(3): pp. 238–47.

144. Newhouse, P., et al., Nicotine treatment of mild cognitive impairment: a 6-month double-blind pilot clinical trial. *Neurology*, 2012. **78**(2): pp. 91–101.

145. Maher, B., Poll results: look who's doping. *Nature*, 2008. **452**(7188): pp. 674–5.

146. Farah, M. J., et al., Neurocognitive enhancement: what can we do and what should we do? *Nat Rev Neurosci*, 2004. **5**(5): pp. 421–5.

147. Vedantam, S., Millions have misused ADHD stimulant drugs, study says, in The Washington Post. 25 February 2006. Accessed 6 November 2012; available from: http://www.washingtonpost.com/wp-dyn/content/article/2006/02/24/AR2006022401773.html.

148. Hillman, C. H., K. I. Erickson, and A. F. Kramer, Be smart, exercise your heart: exercise effects on brain and cognition. *Nature reviews. Neuroscience*, 2008. **9**(1): pp. 58–65.

149. Schlaggar, B. L. and B. D. McCandliss, Development of neural systems for reading. *Annual Review of Neuroscience*, 2007. **30**: pp. 475–503.

150. Boonstra, T. W., et al., Effects of sleep deprivation on neural functioning: an integrative review. *Cellular and Molecular Life Sciences: CMLS*, 2007. **64**(7–8): pp. 934–46.

151. Almeida, S. S., et al., Nutrition and brain function: a multidisciplinary virtual symposium. *Nutritional Neuroscience*, 2002. **5**(5): pp. 311–20.

152. Dodge, T., et al., Judging cheaters: is substance misuse viewed similarly in the athletic and academic domains? *Psychology of addictive behaviors: Journal of the Society of Psychologists in Addictive Behaviors*, 2012. **26**(3): pp.678–82.

153. McCabe, S. E., et al., Non-medical use of prescription stimulants among US college students: prevalence and correlates from a national survey. *Addiction*, 2005. **100**(1): pp. 96–106.

154. Academy of Medical Sciences, Brain science, addiction and drugs in Foresight Brain Science, Addiction and Drugs Project, ed. P. S. G. Horn. 2008, Office of Science and Technology: London.

155. Lennard, N., One in ten takes drugs to study: survey reveals extent of students' medication usage, in Varsity: The Independent Cambridge Student Newspaper, 6 March 2009.

156. Greely, H., et al., Towards responsible use of cognitive-enhancing drugs by the healthy. *Nature*, 2008. **456**(7223): pp. 702–5.

157. Burne, J., Can taking a pill make you brainy?, in Daily Mail: Good Health, 26 December 2007. pp. 64–5.

158. Fukuyama, F., Our Posthuman Future: Consequences of the Biotechnology Revolution. 2002, New York: Farrar, Strauss and Giroux. pp. 256.

159. Academy of Medical Sciences, Human enhancement and the future of work, G. Richardson, chair of steering committee, 2012.

160. Enhancing, not cheating. *Nature*, 2007. **450**(7168): p. 320. Accessed 11 November 2012; available from: http://www.nature.com/nature/journal/v450/n7168/full/450320a.html.

INDEX

INDEX

exposure therapy, *see* flooding
therapy

fight or flight response 44
flooding therapy 144 n.20
fMRI, *see* functional magnetic
resonance imaging
framing 12
in medicine 13
in polls 14
see also Luntz, Frank
frontal lobe, *see* lobe (of brain)
frontotemporal dementia (FTD)
1–2, 64
and decision making 79
and methylphenidate 93
functional magnetic resonance
imaging (fMRI) 33

Gage, Phineas 23–24, 78,
135 n.3, 5
Gall, Franz 21
see also phrenology

hippocampal formation 63,
145 n.24
hippocampus 64, Figure 17
see also hippocampal formation
hot decision 19, 37, 67
computer task 38–9, *see also*
Cambridge Gambling Task
and entrepreneurs 41
see also decision making in mania
and depression
see also orbitofrontal cortex

inequality of access 116
insula 45
intelligence 116
Iowa Gambling Task 77

judgment 4

Kasparov, Garry 47
see also chess
see also Deep Blue

limbic system 46
Lincoln, Abraham 53
Little Albert 139 n.9
lobe (of brain) 45, Figure 12
lobotomy 26–7
and Howard Dully 27
and Walter Freeman 26
Luntz, Frank 13
see also framing

magnetic resonance imaging
(MRI) 30
magnetoencephalography (MEG) 34
mania 55
see also mood disorder
memory
and acetylcholine 89, 90
and Alzheimer's disease 63–4
and attention deficit hyperactivity
disorder 97
and frontotemporal dementia 64
and healthy individuals 94, 99
and the limbic system 46
and nicotine 113
and subarachnoid haemorrhage
(SAH) 87
and traumatic brain injury
(TBI) 93
see also Cambridge
Neuropsychological Test
Automated Battery (CANTAB)
methylphenidate 90
abuse potential 95
and attention deficit hyperactivity
disorder (ADHD) 90, 91
and bipolar disorder 92
cost 149 n.12
and dementia 94